Katharine Beals, Deborah Dahl, Ruth Fink and Marcia Linebarger
Speech and Language Technology for Language Disorders

Speech Technology and Text Mining in Medicine and Health Care

Series Editor
Amy Neustein

Published in the Series

Neustein (Ed.), *Text Mining of Web-Based Medical Content, 2014*
ISBN: 978-1-61451-541-8, e-ISBN 978-1-61451-390-2, e-ISBN (EPUB) 978-1-61451-976-8,
Set-ISBN 978-1-61451-391-9

Neustein (Ed.), *Speech and Automata in Healthcare, 2014*
ISBN 978-1-61451-709-2, e-ISBN 978-1-61451-515-9, e-ISBN (EPUB) 978-1-61451-9607,
Set-ISBN 978-1-61451-516-6

Speech and Language Technology for Language Disorders

Katharine Beals
Deborah Dahl
Ruth Fink
Marcia Linebarger

DE GRUYTER

Authors

Katharine Beals
516 Woodland Terrace
Philadelphia, PA 10194
USA
beals@autism-language-
therapies.com

Deborah Dahl
1820 Gravers Road
Plymouth Meeting, PA 19462
USA
dahl@conversational-
technologies.com

Ruth Fink
60 Township Line Road
Elkins Park, PA 19027
USA
rfink@einstein.edu

Marcia Linebarger
261 Old York Road, Suite 703-B
Jenkintown, PA 19046
USA
linebarger@sentenceshaper.com

MossTalk Words® is a registered trademark of Albert Einstein Healthcare Network. SentenceShaper® is a registered trademark of Psycholinguistic Technologies, Inc. SentenceWeaver™ is a trademark of Autism Language Therapies. All other trademarks mentioned in this book are the properties of their respective owners.

ISBN 978-1-61451-758-0
e-ISBN (PDF) 978-1-61451-645-3
e-ISBN (EPUB) 978-1-61451-925-6
ISSN 2329-5198

Library of Congress Cataloging-in-Publication data
A CIP catalog record for this book has been applied for at the Library of Congress.

Bibliographic information published by the Deutsche Nationalbibliothek
The Deutsche Nationalbibliothek lists this publication in the Deutsche Nationalbibliografie; detailed bibliographic data are available on the Internet at http://dnb.dnb.de.

© 2016 Walter de Gruyter Inc., Boston/Berlin
Cover image: MEHAU KULYK/SCIENCE PHOTO LIBRARY/Agentur Focus
Typesetting: Compuscript Ltd., Shannon, Ireland
Printing and binding: CPI Books GmbH, Leck
♾ Printed on acid-free paper
Printed in Germany

www.degruyter.com

Acknowledgments

We would like to thank the many colleagues who participated in the development and testing of the software discussed in this book and, more importantly, the ideas behind the software.

Katharine Beals would like to thank her son, Jonah Musto, the raison d'être for GrammarTrainer. His ongoing progress motivated each new GrammarTrainer lesson, his clever beta testing fine-tuned its design, and his ultimate achievement motivated its continued development and dissemination. For GrammarTrainer research and development, she would like to thank collaborators at Drexel University, including Felicia Hurewitz, John Dressler, Michel Miller, Obinna Otti, Kimberly Inglot, Joel Rodriguez, Beth Randall, and students in the digital media program, as well as Autism Speaks for a technology grant that funded our initial research. She would also like to thank her husband, David Musto, and her dear friend, Jane Avrich, for their feedback on her parts of the book, and Kyle and Hazel, for their love and support.

Deborah Dahl would like to thank her husband, Richard Schranz, her son Peter Schranz, her daughter, Sarah Schranz-Oliveira, and her son-in-law, Nuno Oliveira, for all their love and support.

The software and theoretical approach described in Chapter 9 reflect many years of discussions with Marcia Linebarger's colleagues in aphasia (Myrna Schwartz, Eleanor Saffran, Rita Berndt, and Denise McCall) and computer science (John Romania, Deborah Dahl, Ted Kantner, and Bjorn Sayers). She is grateful to NIH for funding her professional training and most of the research about the two programs detailed in Chapter 9; and to the many research assistants, clinicians, and people with aphasia who participated in these studies. Finally, she would like to thank her husband, William Garfinkle, and son, Isaac Garfinkle, for their love and support.

Ruth Fink would like to thank her mentor and colleague, Myrna Schwartz, for the many years of support and productive collaborations, her coauthors of MossTalk Words (Myrna Schwartz, Adelyn Brecher, and Mike Montgomery), for creating such a visionary product, Deborah Dahl, for her invaluable guidance and successful implementation of the speech recognition feature, the SLPs who meticulously reviewed and tested the software (Paula Sobel and the speech pathology staff at MossRehab), the research assistants and associates who expertly assisted with these studies (Karen Roy and Amanda Dawson), and all the people with aphasia who participated in our work and gave us valuable feedback. Finally, I thank my husband, Ted, my son Matthew, my daughter and son-in-law, Juliet and Franklin Yates, and my sweet grandsons, Sammy and Zevi for their love and support.

MossTalk Words was developed with partial funding from the McLean Contributionship and MossRehab. Additional funding to disseminate and evaluate the software came from NEC Foundation. The upgrade to speech recognition was funded, in part, under a grant with the Pennsylvania Department of Health. The department specifically disclaims responsibility for any analyses, interpretations, or conclusions. We are further grateful for the funding MTW received from the Albert Einstein Society and assistance and resources made available through the Neuro-Cognitive Rehabilitation Research Network (NCRRN), which was supported by grant no. 1 R34 from the NICHD/NIH.

We would also like to thank several people who helped in the preparation of this book. We would like to thank Amy Neustein, the series editor, for encouraging us to write this book in the first place. We would also like to thank Peter Schranz, editorial assistant, for his invaluable assistance and attention to detail in preparing the citations and bibliography, and finally, we would like to thank Julia Lauterbach at DeGruyter for her help with our endless production questions.

Contents

Deborah Dahl

Katharine Beals, Deborah A. Dahl, Ruth Fink and
Marcia Linebarger

Introduction

Language is a fundamental capability of human beings. It profoundly affects our social relationships, learning, the ability to perform most jobs, and nearly every aspect of everyday life. We celebrate the first words of babies and the early reading achievements of school-age children. We admire eloquent speakers, skilled writers, and people who have mastered several languages. Language pervades human society, and for most of us, producing and understanding language is effortless and almost unnoticed, unless something goes wrong. Although written language and sign languages attest to the fact that not all language is spoken, speech is nevertheless a critical part of communication by language for most people.

For these reasons, speech and language disorders can severely disrupt the lives of those who have the disorders, as well as the lives of their families, friends, and colleagues. Although minor disorders may only amount to an inconvenience, severe disorders can be devastating. Moreover, speech and language disorders are relatively common. According to the National Institute on Deafness and Other Communication Disorders, speech disorders affect 8% to 9% of American children, and 6 to 8 million people in the United States have some form of language impairment (National Institutes of Health, 2010). Thus, finding ways to remediate the disorders as well as help people with these disorders communicate is extremely important. Therapy with professional speech and language pathologists has been the traditional solution, but professional therapy is not always available, it can be expensive even when it is available, and it is not always covered by insurance. In addition, technology has some advantages over humans in that it never gets bored, users need not feel ashamed or embarrassed about their language disorder when talking to a machine, and computers are very good, much better than people, at detailed record keeping, which is important for monitoring improvements over time. However, as useful as software can be, it does not replace speech therapy. In an ideal situation, software should supplement speech therapy with a clinician and can even be integrated into the therapy.

For all of these reasons, many people have become interested in exploring how speech and language technologies such as speech recognition, natural language understanding, dialog processing, and text-to-speech (TTS) could be used to remediate speech and language disorders as well as to provide assistive communication technology for people with these disorders. This interest is also stimulated by recent dramatic increases in the basic capabilities of speech and language technology, the increasing power and decreasing cost of computing devices, and vastly improved development tools, making it much easier to integrate these technologies into applications.

The idea of using technology to address speech and language disorders applies to both remediation and assistive technology. Using technology in remediation can complement or substitute for feedback that a human clinician or family member could provide, or it can simply provide opportunities to practice speech and/or language in a relaxed setting without the time constraints of normal conversation. Speech and language technology in an assistive context can be used to augment or support the user's own capabilities.

This book is about how speech and language technologies can be applied to address language disorders. Although there are many types of language disorders, we will focus specifically on aphasia and on the language disorders associated with autism, because those are our areas of expertise. However, we believe that some of the principles we discuss will apply to software used in addressing other language disorders. We will illustrate how the principles are applied by reviewing examples of software that uses speech and language technologies to address language disorders. In particular, we will describe four software programs in detail. These are (1) GrammarTrainer, which is used by children with autism to improve their sentence construction skills, (2) MossTalk Words®, which is used by adults with aphasia to improve word retrieval skills (3) SentenceShaper®, which helps people with aphasia create speech with their own voices, and (4) Aphasia Therapy System, which provides people with aphasia with detailed feedback on their descriptions of pictures. We have been involved in developing these programs, and we hope that our experiences will prove valuable to readers who are considering using, or even developing, similar software.

Since this book is about applications for speech and language disorders, we will not specifically discuss many potentially valuable applications of speech and language technology with other goals. Some types of applications that we will not discuss are software for normal language development, including reading and foreign language learning; software that addresses sensory and motor problems that affect language, such as deafness and Parkinson's disease; or software that compensates for the effects of normal aging. While we believe that some of the technologies discussed here may well be relevant to these other populations, we focus here on specifically addressing speech and language disorders.

In addition, because this book is about speech and language technologies, we will focus on software that requires the user to actually produce speech or language and that processes the user's speech and language. We also discuss, to a lesser extent, software based on non-linguistic inputs such as pointing (either with a mouse or with a touchscreen); for example, to match a word and a picture. There is some discussion of this approach because point-and-click software can require linguistic processing in order to decide where to point or click. Also, matching a word or sentence to the appropriate picture is relevant because it does require semantic and/or syntactic processing of the word or sentence.

In addition, many of the evaluation principles discussed in Chapter 10 apply to software that uses pointing interaction, so that chapter may also be useful for evaluating pointing-based software.

We discuss both research software and commercial products. Since applying speech and language technologies to language disorders is a relatively new area, many interesting applications have been developed by research teams at universities and hospitals. While in some cases research software may not be as polished or well-supported as commercial software, research software can have unique, cutting-edge capabilities that may be appropriate for specific users. Research software is sometimes available directly from the researchers and may represent advanced, innovative applications that are not yet available commercially. In addition, software developed by research teams is in most cases backed by theoretical principles and controlled experiments in a way that commercial software may not be. On the other hand, applicable research software may not be as easy to find as commercial software. Research software is of particular interest in this book because it is an important tool for learning what does and does not work in the process of developing software.

The best way to apply speech and language technologies to speech and language disorders is not always clear-cut at this early stage. Some areas where the best approach is not always clear are highlighted below.

How to successfully process the speech and language of atypical speakers?

Most speech and language technologies, especially speech recognition, are based on statistical methods that rely heavily on examples of speech and language ("training data") produced by adult native speakers without speech or language disorders. Much of speech recognition's recent success has been due to the availability of enormous amounts of this kind of data. Because of this reliance on general training data disordered speech will not match the training data and will not be recognized as well as speech from someone without a speech or language disorder. Consequently, the system will make more mistakes with disordered speech. The mismatch between what the recognizer expects and what the speaker says can be used as the basis of feedback to encourage the user to improve his/her articulation; however, in some cases, the user has actually said the right thing, but the recognizer has failed to recognize it. Chapter 8, on MossTalk Words, presents some strategies for dealing with speech recognition for atypical speech.

Focused exercises or general practice?

Remediation software can ask the user to perform focused exercises on specific topics or it can provide users with the opportunity to practice speaking and understanding language on topics of their choosing. What are the benefits of each of these strategies, and in what contexts are one or the other or a blend of strategies appropriate?

Different kinds of feedback

If feedback to the user is provided, many choices are possible about the form and detail of the feedback. Feedback is not limited to spoken feedback, but it can be provided by many means, including audio, speech, text, or a variety of forms of graphics. Focused exercises typically require some form of feedback, which can range in specificity from right/wrong to detailed information about the reasons that the user's input was right or wrong. In many cases, however, the user may not need any feedback from the system because the user can tell, either while they are speaking or upon review, if their production was right or wrong. If system feedback is used, then it must depend on the actual processing of speech or language in order for the feedback to be accurate. We will see many examples of different kinds of feedback in this book. At one end of the spectrum, GrammarTrainer and the Aphasia Therapy System provide detailed grammatical feedback. MossTalk Words, in contrast, provides simple right/wrong feedback, and SentenceShaper does not provide any system feedback.

The importance of research

One principle that has become very clear as we have worked on this book is that there is a real need for additional quantitative research aimed at studying the most effective ways to apply speech and language technologies to language disorders. Quantitative research in this area is difficult: funding is limited, it can be difficult to recruit participants, and it can be difficult to assemble the appropriate kinds of interdisciplinary teams that are required to carry out these kinds of studies. We hope that as the tremendous potential for applying speech and language technologies to these very prevalent disorders becomes more widely recognized these problems can be overcome.

The audience

We believe that this book will be of benefit to four audiences. First are application developers, who, we hope, may find these ideas useful as they look for innovative ways that speech and language technology can be used in applications. Second are clinicians who are looking for software that may be of value to their clients. Third are students of speech-language pathology and application development. Finally, we hope that this book will also prove helpful to people with speech and language disorders themselves and their friends and family members, who may be looking for software that can address their needs.

The topics

Chapter 1, written by Deborah Dahl, is a survey of the state of the art in speech and language technologies, including speech recognition, natural language understanding, dialog processing, natural language generation, and TTS. Not all of these have been incorporated into existing therapeutic systems, but even the ones that have not yet been applied may have the potential to be used in innovative ways and new applications.

Following the discussion of technologies, we review applications of speech and language technologies in two general areas, technologies for addressing developmental language disorders and technologies for addressing aphasia.

In Chapter 2, Katharine Beals provides an overview of developmental language disorders, and in Chapter 3, Beals continues with a discussion of technology for assessment and remediation of developmental language disorders.

In Chapter 4, Beals reviews technology for task assessment, classroom accommodation, and communicative assistance of developmental language disorders. Chapter 5 discusses conclusions and caveats about developmental language technology.

Chapter 6, written by Ruth Fink, begins our discussion of aphasia with a review of the different types of naming disorders, followed by Chapter 7, which discusses software for naming disorders.

Chapter 8, by Ruth Fink and Deborah Dahl, discusses MossTalk Words, a program for remediating naming disorders due to aphasia.

Chapter 9, written by Marcia Linebarger, is about the application of speech and language technology to sentence production disorders in aphasia; she discusses Aphasia Therapy System, SentenceShaper, and other software designed to support sentence production in aphasia.

Chapter 10, written by Deborah Dahl, reviews some ways to evaluate software for speech and language disorders.

Chapter 11 summarizes the main themes that emerge from our discussion of these different technologies and populations.

Reference

National Institutes of Health. (2010). *Statistics on voice, speech and language*. Retrieved January 15, 2015, from http://www.nidcd.nih.gov/health/statistics/pages/vsl.aspx

Deborah Dahl

1 Overview of speech and language technologies

Abstract: This chapter provides a technical overview and description of the state of the art for current speech and language processing technologies. It focuses on the technologies that have been particularly useful in assistive and remediative applications for people with speech and language disorders. The major technologies discussed include speech recognition, natural language processing, dialog management, and text to speech. The chapter also briefly reviews other related technologies such as avatars, text simplification and natural language generation.

1.1 Introduction to speech and language technologies

Speech and language technologies are technologies that allow computers to perform some of the functions of human linguistic communication – including recognizing and understanding speech, reading text out loud, and engaging in a conversation. Although human abilities to communicate with each other far outstrip the current state of the art in speech and language technologies, the technologies are progressing rapidly and are certainly suitable for application to specific, well-defined problems. There will not be a single, all-encompassing, spoken language understanding system that can be applied to every situation any time soon, but if we look at specific contexts and needs, there very well may be ways that these technologies in their current state can be extremely helpful.

The technologies that will be discussed in this chapter do not in most cases serve those with speech and language disorders directly. Rather, these technologies are more typically deployed to supply speech- and language-processing capabilities as part of applications that, in turn, are specifically dedicated to these populations.

The entire field of speech and language technologies is very broad and can be broken down into many very specialized technologies. We will focus here on the subset of speech and language technologies that show particular promise for use in addressing language disorders. The main focus will be on speech recognition (sometimes also called speech-to-text), natural language understanding, and dialog systems. However, other emerging technologies such as text simplification and natural language generation can potentially play a role in addressing speech and language disorders, so these technologies will also be mentioned briefly.

We will primarily be concerned with applications of the technologies in assistive and remediation situations. However, some of the technologies can also be applied toward other goals, for example, automatic assessment of users' capabilities and automatic logging and record keeping for clinical and research purposes. We will also touch on these types of applications.

We will focus in this chapter on the technologies themselves, regardless of how they are used in specific applications or research projects, noting that in almost every case, basic technologies will be combined with other software (and hardware) to create specific applications.

Because speech and language technologies are modeled on human capabilities, it is useful to discuss them in the context of a complete system that models a human conversational participant; that is, an interactive dialog system. Conversations between people go back and forth between the conversational participants, each participant speaking and listening at different times. This back-and-forth pattern is called *turn-taking*, and each speaker's contribution is called a *turn*. In the majority of normal conversations, each turn is more or less related to the previous speaker's turn. Thus, participating in a human-human conversation requires skills in listening, understanding, deciding what to say, composing an appropriate response, and speaking. These skills are mirrored in the technologies that are used to build spoken dialog systems: speech recognition, natural language understanding, dialog management, natural language generation, and text-to-speech (TTS). For people with speech and language disorders, then, these separate technologies can potentially be applied to compensate for disorders that affect each of these skills.

Figure 1.1 is an example of a complete interactive dialog system. A user speaks or types to the system, then the natural language understanding component processes the user's input and represents the input in a structured way so that it can be used by a computer. The dialog management component acts on the

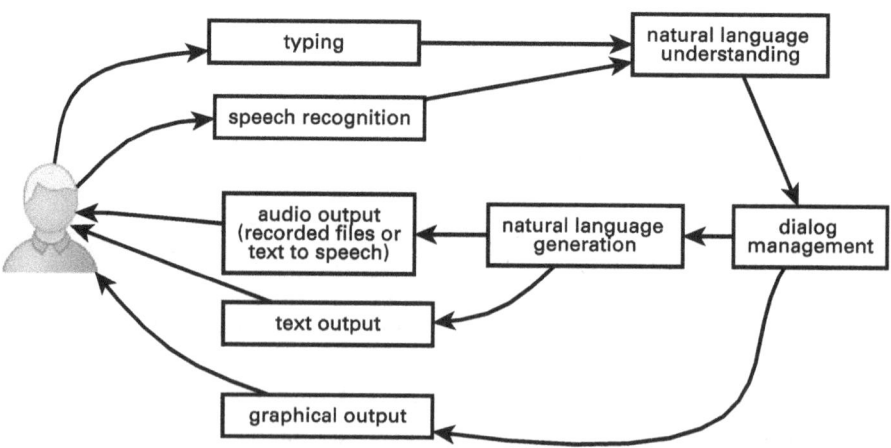

Fig. 1.1: Complete interactive dialog system.

user's input and decides what to do next. The next action might be some kind of response to the user, interaction with the user's environment, or feedback to the user on their input. Unlike conversations between people, where the responses will almost always be linguistic, responses in an interactive dialog system can also be in the form of displayed text or graphics.

As we will see in the rest of this book, these technologies can be mixed and matched in a variety of ways in different applications to address different remediation or assistive goals. As an example, Fig. 1.2 shows a simpler version of a spoken dialog system, designed to provide the user with feedback on their speech or on individual spoken words. It does not attempt to provide the user with feedback on language, so it does not require a natural language understanding component. Rather, speech is recognized, and the recognized speech is sent to the

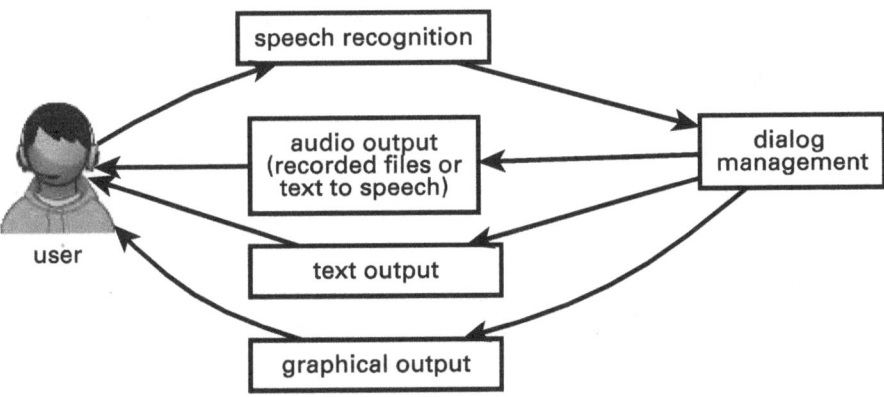

Fig. 1.2: Speech/lexical feedback components.

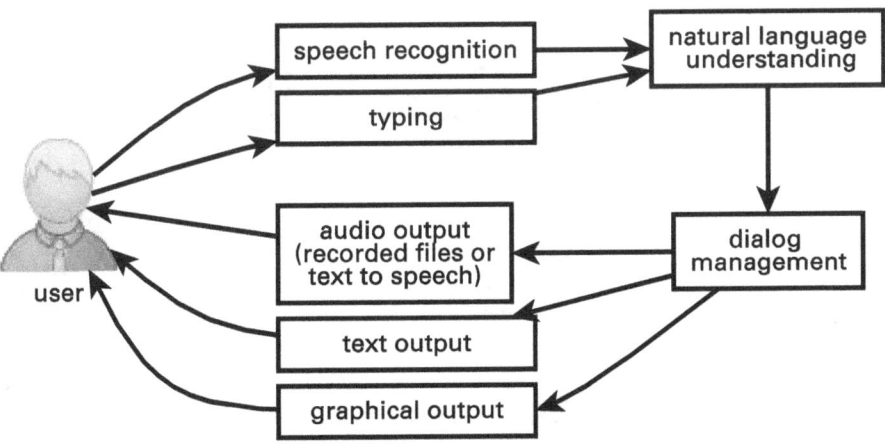

Fig. 1.3: System for language/grammar feedback.

dialog management component, which then provides the user with feedback in the form of text audio output and graphical output. This system describes the general structure of MossTalk Words, discussed in Chapter 8.

As another example, a system designed to provide the user only with feedback on their language would look more like the system shown in Fig. 1.3. Here the user speaks or types to the system with the intention of producing a more or less complete sentence. This kind of system is focused on providing feedback to the user on their language; although speech would be an option for input, typed input is also possible with this kind of system, if that is appropriate for the application and for the users. GrammarTrainer, an application for helping users with autism improve their grammar, discussed in Chapter 3, is a system of this kind. Users interact with GrammarTrainer with typed input.

Another system with a similar organization is the Aphasia Therapy System discussed in Chapter 9, for users with aphasia, which analyzes users spoken language and provides detailed feedback on their productions.

Another type of organization is shown in Fig. 1.4. This system allows the user to record short pieces of speech and assemble them into longer spoken sentences or series of sentences. An example of this type of system is SentenceShaper®, discussed in Chapter 8. The dialog manager in this case is simply the software that reacts to the user's commands to record and play back speech at different levels.

The next few sections will discuss in more detail the individual technologies that comprise these systems. This material can be treated as background reading. It is useful in understanding the technologies that can be applied to speech and language disorders and their limitations, especially for developers, but readers can skip over the rest of this chapter if they are not interested in the details of the underlying technologies.

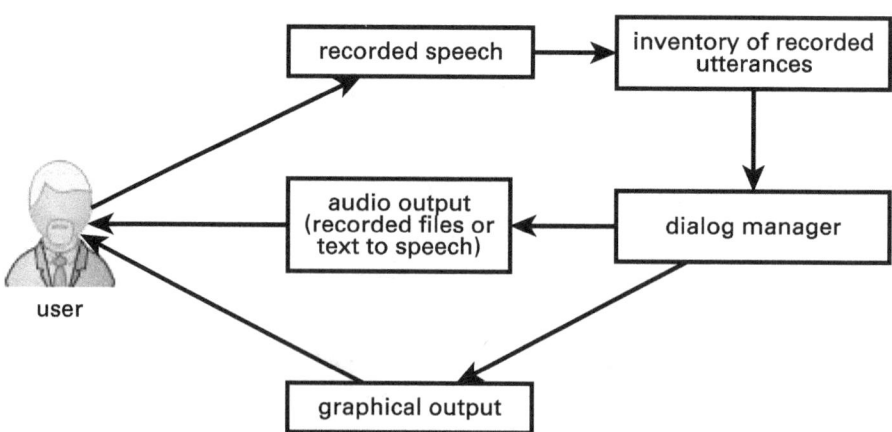

Fig. 1.4: System for user-initiated control and playback of user utterances.

1.2 Speech recognition

1.2.1 What is speech recognition?

Speech recognition is the technology that enables a computer to turn speech into written language. It is sometimes called "speech-to-text". More technically, speech recognition is referred to as automatic speech recognition to distinguish it from human speech recognition. One way to think of a speech recognizer is as the software counterpart of a human stenographer or transcriptionist. The speech recognizer simply records the words that it hears, without attempting to understand them.

Speech recognition starts with capturing speech and converting it from sound, which is physically a sequence of rapid changes in air pressure, into an electrical signal that mirrors the sound, the *waveform*, through the use of a microphone. Perhaps surprisingly, the waveforms for what we perceive as a sequence of words do not include physical gaps corresponding to what we perceive as word boundaries. There are rarely silences between words in actual speech, and conversely, there can be silences in the middle of words that we do not perceive as silence. In addition, the same sounds can be spoken in many different ways, even though they sound to human listeners like the same sound. In addition to the speaker's words, many additional factors can affect the actual physical sounds of speech. These include the speaker's accent, the speaker's age, how clearly the speech is articulated, how rapid it is, and whether the conversation is casual or formal. In addition, in the real world, speech will inevitably be mixed in with other sounds in the environment, such as noise, music, and speech from other people. One of the most difficult problems today in speech recognition research is separating the speech that a system is interested in from other sounds in the environment, particularly from other speech. For all of these reasons, the technologies behind the process of converting sounds to written words are very complex.

As an example, Fig. 1.5 shows the waveform for the word "speech" spoken three times, with the sounds mapped to the parts of the waveform to which they correspond. Distance from the middle indicates the amount of energy in the signal at that point. Note that none of these look exactly the same, even though they were spoken by the same person at almost the same time. We can also see

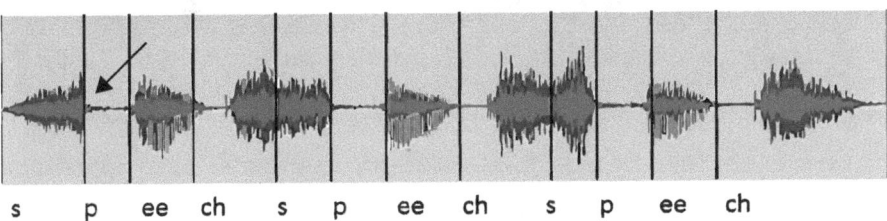

Fig. 1.5: Speech waveform for the word "speech" spoken three times.

that the "ch" at the end of each "speech" merges into the "s" at the beginning of the next word without any actual silence (as indicated by a flat line in the waveform). Also note that the "p's" and the "ch's" each contain a brief introductory silence, pointed to by the arrow for the first "p", that we do not hear as a silence.

The following discussion presents a very high level overview of how today's speech recognition technology works. Speech recognition is the process of trying to match waveforms, as shown in Fig. 1.5, which are highly variable, to the sounds and words of a language. Because of the variable nature of the waveforms, the process of speech recognition is heavily statistical, relying on large amounts of previously transcribed speech, which provides examples of how sounds (the signal) match up to the words of a language. Basically, the recognizer is trying to find the best match between the signal and the words of the language, but mistakes, or misrecognitions, are very possible, particularly when the speech occurs under challenging conditions that make it harder to hear.

The next task in speech recognition is to analyze the waveform into its component frequencies. Speech, like all sounds, can be broken down into a combination of frequencies, referring to different rates of vibration in the sound. Frequencies are measured in terms of cycles per second, or hertz (Hz). We perceive lower frequencies as lower-pitched sounds and higher frequencies as higher-pitched sounds. The energy present in the signal at different frequencies is referred to as the *spectrum*.

The spectrum is more useful in speech recognition than the waveform because it shows more clearly the amount of energy present at different frequencies at each point in time. This energy is very diagnostic of the specific speech sounds (phonemes) that are being spoken.

The spectrum in Fig. 1.6 shows the word "speech" spoken three times. Time is shown on the horizontal axis, the frequencies of the different components of the signal are shown on the vertical axis, and the darkness and lightness indicates the amount of energy present in the signal at each frequency at each point in time. For example, for the three occurrences of the vowel "ee" in the three repetitions of

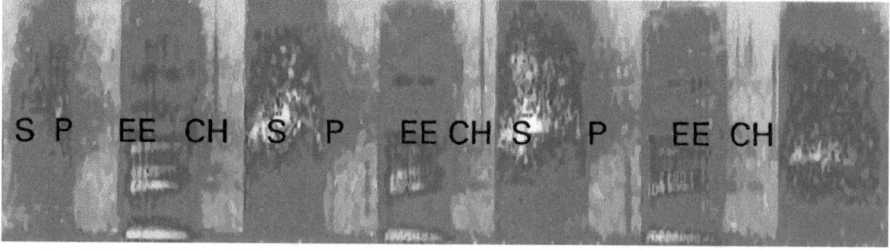

Fig. 1.6: Spectrum of the word "speech" spoken three times, showing the approximate location of the speech sounds.

the word "speech", we can see bands of high energy, shown in white, continuing through the vowel. These bands, called *formants*, are characteristic of vowels. Less energetic regions are shown in a darker gray, and low-energy regions are shown in light gray. There is some noise present throughout the signal, shown by the diffuse light gray areas.

The process of speech recognition involves looking at the properties, or *acoustic features*, of very short time slices, on the order of a few milliseconds, in the spectrum. The goal is to identify the actual speech sounds present in the signal. There are many types of acoustic features that can be used, including the amount of energy present at different frequencies, the relative duration of the sound, and dynamic changes in the frequency distribution of the sound. Because so many speech sounds are similar, just taking into account the acoustic features rarely defines exactly which sound was spoken. This means that for a particular waveform, there will be many alterative hypotheses about what sounds might have occurred at each point in time. To narrow down these hypotheses, the recognizer also takes into account a *language model* that describes the expected order of words in the spoken language. For example, a spoken sequence like "the ball is under the table" is much more probable than "under ball table the the is". If the acoustic evidence is consistent with both sequences, the recognizer will choose the more probable sequence, "the ball is under the table" as its result, or *hypothesis*. Different kinds of language models are appropriate for different applications of speech recognition; we will discuss these in more detail below.

1.2.2 Additional information – *confidence* and *nbest*

Besides the final, most probable, hypothesis about a sequence of words, recognizers also typically provide some additional information that can be used in applications but is usually not visible to end users. Two important examples of this kind of additional information are *confidence* and *nbest* results. As we said earlier, speech recognition is a statistical process, which means it does not provide a hard and fast yes-or-no answer to the question of what the true recognition result is for a particular utterance. Confidence is a number, usually between 0 and 1, that represents the recognizer's level of certainty that the result it provided was correct. The closer the confidence is to 1, the more certain the recognizer is of the result. This is useful because an application that receives the results from the speech recognizer can choose to treat high- and low-confidence results differently. For example, the application might ask a user to explicitly confirm a relatively low-confidence result, or it may even ignore a very low-confidence result, depending on the purpose of the application.

Similarly, although the recognizer will deliver a top choice for the recognition result, there may also be other alternative possibilities – ones with lower confidences than the top choice. These alternative possibilities are called the *nbest list*. An application might look at the *nbest list* and, if the alternatives are similar to each other in confidence, ask the user to pick one of them. For example, a user could say, "The weather is very nice today", but the top recognition result might be "The weather's very nice today". If the user wants to correct that, the recognizer might offer alternative hypotheses from the *nbest list* for "weather's" such as "weathers'", "weather is", or even "withers".

1.2.3 Types of language models

As we said earlier, speech recognition systems are constrained by language models, which represent information about the possible sequences of words that are expected in utterances in a language. Two general types of language model have been used in speech recognition.

1.2.3.1 Grammar-based language models

The first type of language model is a grammar, which is a full specification of all the sequences of words (or *utterances*) that can be recognized by the speech recognizer. Rather than a simple list of all the possible sequences of words, grammars are normally written in special shorthands that collapse multiple utterances in a single rule. Some common rule formats are the World Wide Web Consortium's Speech Recognition Grammar Specification (SRGS) (W3C 2004), the Java Speech Grammar Format (JSGF), and Nuance's GSL. (These are technically special types of grammars, called context-free grammars, or CFGs.)

Figure 1.7 shows a very simplified grammar that specifies only a few sentences, such as "the boy fed the cat" and "the girl played with the dog". Sentences in this grammar consist of a subject, followed by a verb, followed by an object. A vertical

Sentence → Subject Verb Object

Subject → the boy | the girl

Verb → fed | played with

Object → the cat | the dog

Fig. 1.7: A simple grammar.

line represents a choice, so the subject could either be "the boy" or "the girl". This is a very simple grammar and is only an example for illustrating the concept. Real speech recognition grammars are usually much more complex and use special syntaxes that are meaningful to the speech recognizer, such as those listed above.

Grammar-based language models are very strict and are most useful in contexts where the speech recognition task is very difficult; for example, they are typically used in systems that must recognize speech over landline telephones. The problem with grammar-based language models in most applications is that they are very unforgiving of any deviations from the expected order of words. If a sequence of words occurs in the user's speech that is not anticipated in the grammar, the recognizer will either misrecognize the utterance as something that is actually in the grammar or alternatively, it will fail to recognize anything at all. This can be very frustrating for users, who often find it quite difficult to figure out what the system expects, especially if the application uses only speech and does not include a graphical component that can display options. Of course, the strictness of a grammar-based language model is a benefit if the goal of speech recognition is to make certain that the speaker uses an exact phrase. But this can only be done if the speaker knows what the exact required phrase is and pronounces it correctly. In some applications, this is indeed the case. Examples of this type of application are "read-aloud" applications that help people practice reading (Williams, Nix & Fairweather 2000; Kartal 2006; Scientific Learning 2015). In that type of application, the required phrase is simply the text presented to the user for reading. If the user does not say the expected phrase and speech recognition fails, that is a desirable outcome for this application. Similarly, an application for people with naming disorders can present the user with a picture and a strict grammar-based recognizer can be used to decide if the user has said the right word, correctly naming the picture. This technique is used in MossTalk Words®, discussed in detail in Chapter 8.

On the other hand, if the speaker has no way of knowing what the required phrase is, he or she can become quite frustrated in trying to figure out what to say. Even more frustrating for the speaker is when he or she does say what the system expects, but the recognizer fails to recognize it for some other reason – poor articulation due to a speech disorder, noise, or an unexpected accent, for example.

1.2.3.2 Statistical language models

The other type of language model used with speech recognition is a statistical language model (SLM). This approach is much more forgiving of unexpected inputs.

This type of model is increasingly becoming more common as the underlying accuracy of basic speech recognition technology increases. A statistical model is based on not rules, but on an analysis of large amounts of text. This analysis, called *training*, discovers the probability of word sequences in the text and uses those probabilities in the speech recognition process. For example, the sequence "it it the" is very unlikely to occur in normal text. In contrast, a sequence of "the" followed by an adjective or noun is much more likely. However, because the sequences of words are probabilistic, a recognizer using an SLM will not completely rule anything out; it will simply prefer the more likely sequences of words over the less likely sequences of words. Statistical models are most commonly used in applications for which it would be extremely difficult to develop a grammar, for example, dictation or web search applications, since the order of the words that might be used in dictation or web search is very hard to predict. Speech recognizers for dictation and web search include Dragon Naturally Speaking™ from Nuance, Windows Speech Recognition, Google voice search, Bing voice search, and the speech recognition used on iOS devices. They are useful for creating text and thus can help people with language disorders or motor problems that make writing difficult.

A variation of the SLM that is more constrained than a completely open dictation model is one that is specific to a particular application and is custom-built for that application by data collected from users using the application. Examples of application-specific SLMs are SLMs built for telephone applications like telephone banking applications or technical troubleshooting applications. This type of statistical model provides more constraint (and consequently will be more accurate) than a completely open dictation model but it is much less constrained than a grammar-based approach. However, developing an application-specific SLM is the most expensive approach to using speech recognition in an application, since it requires collecting and annotating a large number of utterances on the topic of the application. This is usually not feasible except for large commercial call center deployments.

Applications for users with speech and language disorders that use speech recognition are typically based on either grammars or open dictation technology, not application-specific SLMs. This is probably due to a combination of the expense of creating these types of systems and the difficulty of finding developers who can develop application-specific SLMs.

1.2.4 When can speech recognition help?

Speech recognition can be used to help people with speech and language disorders in a variety of ways.

1. Speech recognition can supplement human speech and language pathologists in remediation situations by listening to the user's speech and reacting to it – for example, by giving the user feedback on the correctness of his or

her speech. Speech recognition systems are by no means as accurate as a human therapist, but speech recognition applications are less expensive and more available than speech and language pathologists, particularly if the application is installed in the user's home or on a mobile device.

2. Speech recognition can help users create text hands-free if they can speak better than they can write.
3. For users who can read but not understand speech (for example, the hearing-impaired), speech recognition technology can be used as an assistive technology. Someone else who is trying to communicate with the user can speak to the application, which can then show the user the text.
4. Speech recognition can be used to support practice for someone with articulation difficulties. At first, the recognizer may have difficulty understanding the user's speech, and this failure to understand can provide feedback to the user. As the user's articulation improves, the speech recognizer will be better able to recognize his or her words as they are pronounced more accurately.

Later chapters will expand on these ideas in detail.

1.2.5 Limits of current technology

Although speech recognition works very well in certain specific applications, for example, desktop dictation or mobile web search, there are many kinds of speech that are still challenging for current recognizers. Speech that occurs in noisy environments or speech that comes from speakers with unexpected accents or disordered speech, or from children, or from multiple simultaneous speakers is recognized less well. This is because the speech signal that is presented to the recognizer at runtime does not bear a very strong resemblance (in terms of acoustic features) to the signals with which it was originally trained. This makes the speech recognition task more difficult.

Environmental noise will probably be less of an issue in remediation applications because speech therapy is more likely to take place in relatively predictable environments, such as a clinic, (although this may not always be the case if the remediation software is being used in a home environment). In contrast, an assistive device that uses speech recognition in unpredictable environments will suffer from a decrease in speech recognition accuracy to a greater or lesser extent, depending on the severity of the environment. Cars, train stations, noisy restaurants, and most outdoor settings all present challenging environments to speech recognition technology. This points to the importance of evaluating assistive devices that use speech recognition in the normal environment in which they will be used. An application that works well in a quiet room may be unusable outdoors or in a car.

Children's speech is also relatively difficult to recognize, especially younger children's speech. This is due to several factors, including the fact that most speech recognizers are developed based on adult speech, and also because some children, especially younger children, have not yet fully acquired the ability to form the sounds in their language. As a consequence, their speech does not sound like the kind of speech the recognizer was expecting. This concern applies even more to disordered speech, whether from children or from adults. Some recent work has been done on speech recognition for children's speech, which should improve the technology available for applications as it becomes commercialized (see, for example, Shivakumar, Potamianos, Lee & Narayanan 2014).

Some speech and language disorders are characterized by abnormal intonation, or *prosody*. Unfortunately, speech recognition research has largely focused on recognizing words, and has done relatively little work on recognizing intonation. In fact, most speech recognition software explicitly ignores prosody in order to focus on creating written text. Although there are exceptions in the research literature (Panttaja 1988; Vicsi & Szaszák 2010), this means that technologies for speech and language disorders that involve problems with intonation are not yet available. However, some research has been done on tools that might be used in a system that provides feedback on prosody (for example, Vicsi & Szaszák 2010).

1.2.6 Availability of speech recognition technology

Speech recognition technology is widely available and can be accessed in many different ways. It is built into current desktop computers and mobile devices and can be accessed programmatically in most cases by developers who would like to integrate it into applications. Windows Speech Recognition, for example, can be used with both grammars and with dictation on Windows computers. Nuance is a major vendor of paid speech recognition technology, including the Dragon family of speech recognizers for desktop and mobile applications.

IBM, Nuance, and Wit.ai (Facebook) have made their speech technology available as web services. Google's speech recognition is accessible from Android devices and from the Chrome browser. Microsoft Windows speech recognizer is available for integration with desktop applications, and Microsoft also provides the ability to integrate speech into apps for Windows 8 and Windows Phone. iSpeech provides a cross-platform SDK for mobile and desktop applications. The Sphinx family of speech recognizers from Carnegie-Mellon University is the best-known open-source recognition system (Lee 1989; The CMU Sphinx Group 2009), although using it requires some expertise in speech recognition technology.

1.3 Natural language understanding

The next technology that we will discuss is natural language understanding. While speech recognition converts spoken language to written text, natural language understanding recognizes the structure and meaning of a written text.

1.3.1 What is natural language understanding?

Natural language understanding is a set of technologies for converting unstructured natural speech and text into representations of their meaning and structure that can be interpreted by a computer to do something.

1.3.2 Analyzing meaning

Of course, "meaning" is a qualitative word, but in the case of natural language understanding technology, *meaning* usually refers to a structured format that can be comprehended or acted upon by a computer. Figure 1.8 shows an example of how an unstructured utterance, "I want to go from Chicago to New York on August 17 in the early afternoon on United", can be represented in a structured format, consisting of *slots* ("destination" and "departure date") and *values*, such as "New York" and "August 17". In theory, it might be useful to some users to see their speech converted to a structure like the one in Fig. 1.8. Although we are not aware of any specific applications for people with language disorders that display structured meaning, it is possible that converting text or speech to a structured representation and presenting it to the user could be useful in several ways. In an assistive context, it might be helpful for people who have problems comprehending written or spoken language. In a remediation context, it might be useful for helping people practice producing spoken or written language by showing them how their utterances would be represented in a structured way, even potentially flagging duplicate or missing information.

I want to go from Chicago to New York on August 17 in the early afternoon on United

Structured Format – airline reservation
      Destination: New York
      Departure city: Chicago
      Departure date: August 17
      Departure time: early afternoon
      Airline: United

Fig. 1.8: Natural language understanding: creating a structured format from unstructured language.

How is a representation such as the one in Fig. 1.8 produced? Natural language understanding is traditionally conceptualized as a series of tasks in which each task reveals some level of structure within the utterance. The natural-language-processing technology maps one level of structure into another level, building on each level, with the final level being the "meaning" of the utterance. A concrete example would be the following. Starting with text, the first step is to analyze the words to separate root words and the suffixes that indicate grammatical functions, like "-ed", or "-s". This converts words like "walked" into "walk+ed", or "walk+past". Words are also looked up in a dictionary at this initial stage.

In some systems, another process then takes place called *part of speech tagging*. This assigns the most probable part of speech (noun, verb, adjective, adverb, and so on) to each word. This is useful because many words, in isolation, could belong to any of several different parts of speech.

The results of part of speech tagging for one sentence are shown in Tab. 1.1.[1] Although part of speech tagging itself may not have any direct applications to assistive

Tab. 1.1: Part of speech tags for "I want to go from Chicago to New York on August 17 in the afternoon on United".

Word	Part of speech
I	Personal pronoun
want	Past tense verb
to	Infinitive marker
go	Infinitive verb
from	Preposition
Chicago	Proper noun
to	Preposition
New	Proper noun
York	Proper noun
on	Preposition
August	Proper noun
17th	Ordinal number
in	Preposition
the	Article
early	Adjective
afternoon	Common noun
on	Preposition
United	Proper noun

---

[1] This analysis was produced by the OpenNLP natural language processing system. The set of parts of speech is the one used in the Penn Treebank, which is more detailed than traditional parts of speech and better for computer processing.

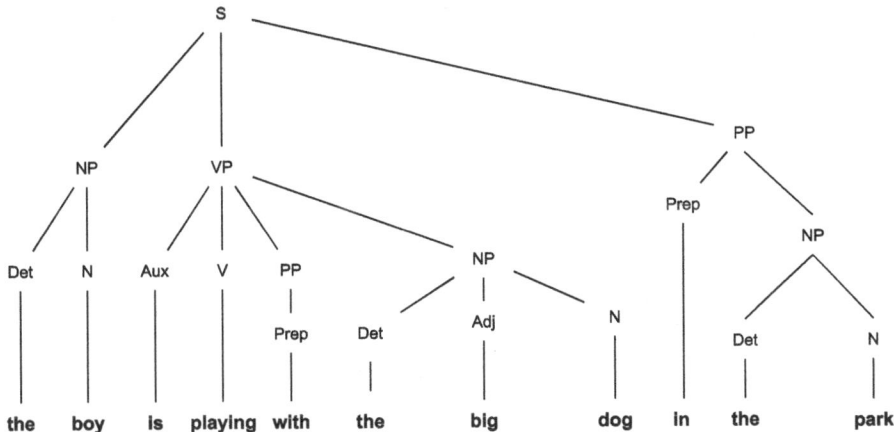

Fig. 1.9: Syntactic parse tree.

and therapeutic software itself, it may have potential for use in applications for assisting therapists in analyzing the speech and text produced by their clients (for example, looking at ratios of different parts of speech).

The next stage of structure, which is built on the results of dictionary lookup and part of speech tagging, is *syntactic analysis*, or *parsing*. The goal of syntactic analysis is to represent the relationships among the words and phrases of the sentence. In most sentences, this will be a hierarchical structure with several layers of representation, or parse tree, as shown in Fig. 1.9. The words are grouped into phrases, such as the noun phrase (NP) "the boy", which are in turn grouped into larger phrases that combine to form a sentence. Syntactic analysis is based on grammars that are similar to, but more complex than, speech grammars such as the one shown in Fig. 1.7.

The syntactic parse tree represents the organization of the structure of the sentence, independently of its meaning. Following syntactic analysis, the next step is to analyze the syntactic parse tree to determine the relationships among the words and phrases of the sentence that have to do with meaning (*semantic analysis*). Semantic analysis is based on additional rules that map the syntactic structures such as "subject", "direct object", etc. into semantic concepts. For example, in Fig. 1.10, the subject of the sentence, "the boy" is mapped to the *semantic role* of *actor*, that is, the one who performs the action described by the sentence. Since "the boy is playing with the dog" is very close in meaning in this example to "the boy and the dog played" or "the dog is playing with the boy", the dog can be described as a *co-actor*. Finally, "the park" can be assigned the semantic role of *location* because that is where the playing is being done. This results in a structured meaning representation such as that shown in Fig. 1.10,

The boy is playing with the big dog in the park

Actor: boy
Action: playing
Co-actor: dog
Location: park

Fig. 1.10: Structured format for "the boy is playing with the big dog in the park".

and in a more detailed way, relating the semantic analysis to the syntactic analysis, in Fig. 1.11.

There are many computational techniques that have been used in the field of natural language processing to produce these kinds of analyses, the details of which go far beyond the scope of this book. However, it is worth noting that many approaches do not attempt to create explicit representations of all the linguistic levels described above. In particular, they do not build a *meaning-independent*, general syntactic analysis of a text or utterance such as the one shown in rather, their approach is to attempt to map the words to meanings more directly.

This direct approach is motivated by the need for some applications to interpret utterances for which a full syntactic parse according to a grammar is not possible – for example, an utterance that includes errors or false starts, which are very common in speech, especially the speech of individuals with speech and language disorders. Skipping the explicit syntactic analysis stage is possible if the goal of the system is simply to understand the user, which is the case for most general purpose applications. On the other hand, if the goal of the system in a therapy context is to assist users in improving their grammar, overlooking syntactic errors is not at all what the system needs to do. In that case, attempting to construct a full syntactic analysis in order to identify grammatical errors could be very useful.

The issue of whether to create a full syntactic analysis is one case of a larger question that all speech applications must address: how "forgiving" the system should be of various types of errors. If the system ignores syntax, and only looks for specific words or phrases, it will automatically ignore grammatical errors. But even if it does compute syntactic analyses, it must choose which kinds of syntactic errors to ignore and which kinds of errors to call to the attention of the user.

One example of a strict-vs.-forgiving approach toward phonological errors, MossTalk Words (which will be discussed in Chapter 8 in detail) allows the user or clinician to set the system to accept phonological errors in speech or to generally accept any incorrect pronunciation (by lowering the recognizer's confidence threshold), as shown in Fig. 1.12, making the application more forgiving. A more forgiving system will accept more utterances, some of which should be accepted, but some of which should not. A human clinician will be able to make more

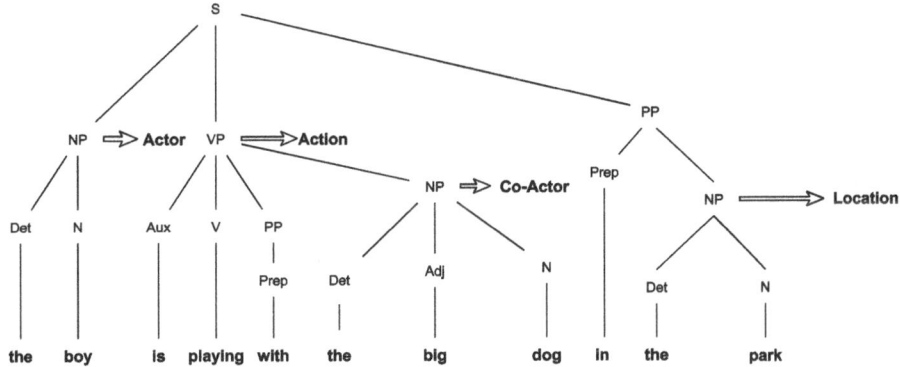

Fig. 1.11: Semantic analysis.

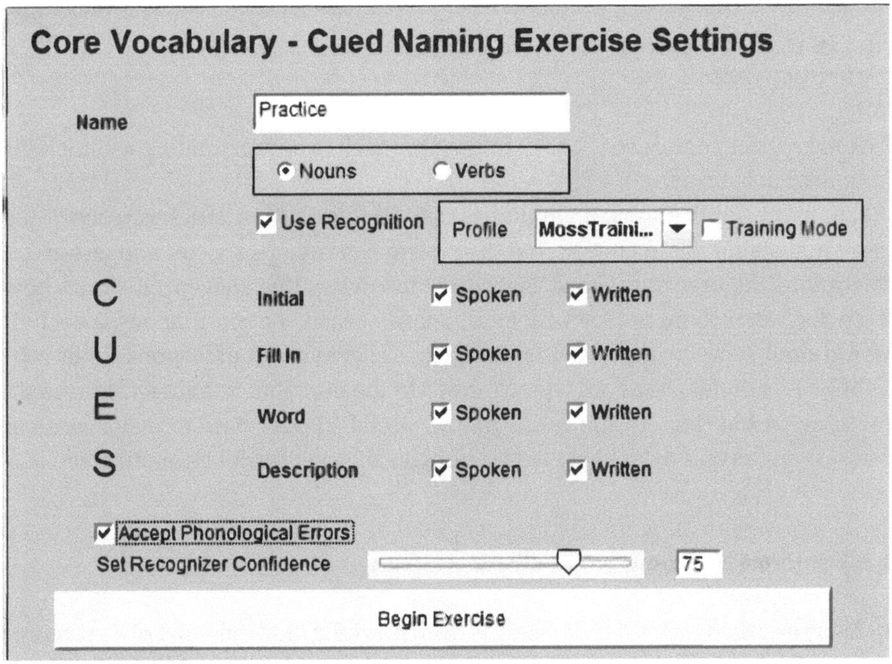

Core Vocabulary - Cued Naming Exercise Settings

Name: Practice

⦿ Nouns ○ Verbs

☑ Use Recognition   Profile MossTraini... ▼ ☐ Training Mode

C   Initial   ☑ Spoken   ☑ Written

U   Fill In   ☑ Spoken   ☑ Written

E   Word   ☑ Spoken   ☑ Written

S   Description   ☑ Spoken   ☑ Written

☑ Accept Phonological Errors
Set Recognizer Confidence   ━━━━━━━◇━━━━   75

Begin Exercise

Fig. 1.12: MossTalk Words exercise setup screen.

fine-grained distinctions between errors and correct pronunciations, but the system will often have to operate in situations where a clinitian is not available. Moreover, a human clinician can decide, based on the goals of therapy, whether to draw the client's attention to an articulation error or to focus on the meaning of what the user says. Setting the parameters for "accept phonological errors" and

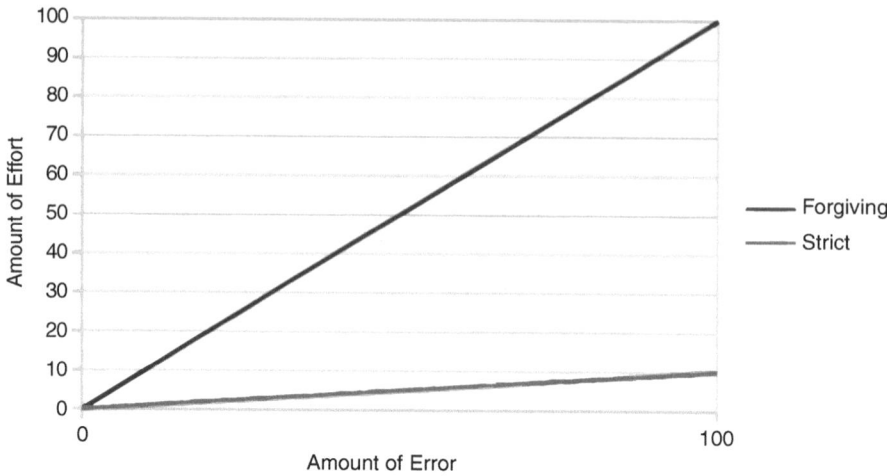

Fig. 1.13: Effort expended by the system to understand errorful input with strict and forgiving systems.

"set recognizer confidence" are a simple approach to approximating a clinician's judgment in software.

In many applications, it would be useful if forgiving vs. strict were available as an adjustable parameter, so that the system can become stricter and less error-tolerant as the user progresses. Figure 1.13 illustrates this concept. It shows how a strict system would not try very hard to make sense out of erroneous speech; it would simply give up and provide feedback, either as a lack of response or by providing more detail about the type of error. On the other hand, a forgiving system, focusing on figuring out the user's intent, would try very hard to make sense of errorful inputs and most likely would not give the user feedback about errors.

1.3.3 Information about intermediate structure

In many cases, the goal of processing is to arrive at the final meaning of a sentence, making the best of any errors. In other systems, the goal is to give the user feedback on errors. In these applications, the goal is not so much to find the final meaning of an utterance but to identify some of the grammatical and lexical structures that contribute to the meaning. Of course, it is unlikely that the actual syntactic analysis (as shown in the tree in Fig. 1.9) would be useful on its own to a non-expert; however, it can potentially be converted by a therapeutic program into meaningful feedback to a user who has difficulty producing full sentences. For example, the Aphasia Therapy System (to be discussed in Chapter 9) provides visual feedback about which verb arguments have been correctly expressed in sentences spoken by the user. Syntactic analysis might also be useful as a component in assessment or diagnostic tools for researchers or clinicians who would like to be able to automatically quantify (without manual coding) the degree of structure in utterances produced by clients.

1.3.4 Converting language to action

Once the user's speech has been understood and represented in a structured form, it can be used to perform actions. Actions can be almost anything – controlling the environment, getting information from the Internet, conversing with the user, or almost anything that can be accomplished through speaking, providing there is a way for the action to be executed. Thus, the failure to perform an action correctly, based on a verbal command, can be a form of indirect but often entertaining feedback on the user's use of the verbal command. For example, if the user is playing a voice-controlled game and says, "move the ball up", then, if the system correctly understands the user, the ball should move up. If the ball does not move up, or moves somewhere else, that would be a form of feedback that the user's command was not understood.

An interesting example of how interpreting language and performing an action can provide feedback is Wordseye, an application that generates an image from a natural language description. As an example, Wordseye generated the image in Fig. 1.14 from the natural language description "The cat is light gray. The cat is on top of the ball. A small white dog is next to the cat. A dark gray cube is next to the dog. The cube is six inches high". Wordseye could be used as a tool

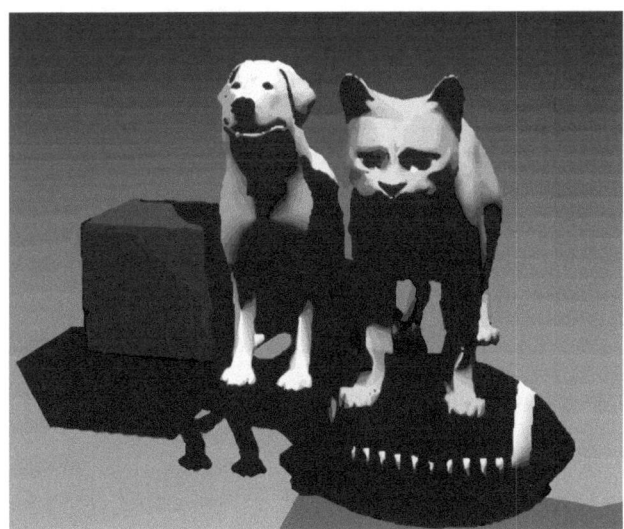

Fig. 1.14: Wordseye image.

for practicing language because the feedback (getting the picture that the user wanted) is interesting and even failures are entertaining.

1.3.5 Limits of current natural language understanding systems

For systems designed to extract linguistic structure from an utterance or text, there are two major limitations in the current technologies. First, extracting structure requires a grammar and dictionary. Although grammatical coverage of English, other major European languages, and major Asian languages is fairly complete, coverage is not available for many languages. This situation should improve with time as techniques for developing grammars and dictionaries become more efficient. The second limitation of current technologies is that, because they are not precise technologies, it is possible for these systems to make errors. Errors are more likely to occur in some parts of the analysis than others. For example, because syntactic analysis is a more difficult task than part of speech tagging, more errors are likely to occur with syntactic structural analysis tasks than with part of speech tagging. The number of errors in syntactic analysis will increase as the length and complexity of the input sentences increase. Consequently, users of these technologies, or applications based on these technologies, will need to be aware of the possibility of analytical errors.

Systems that are designed to extract meaning directly, rather than through the construction of intermediate levels of syntactic structure, suffer from their own limitations. Most importantly, they work best in relatively closed domains. The example in Fig. 1.8 shows a closed domain, airline reservations. Given a closed context or domain, the system is able to assume that all utterances directed to it are relevant to that context. That is why, for example, a natural-language-processing system of this kind can classify "New York" as a "destination". In the closed context of airline reservations, a city name can mean only a destination or departure city. In contrast, in an open domain, the system can only know general information, for example, that Chicago is a city. In fact, in other contexts "Chicago" might not even refer to the city, it could, for example, refer to a sports team. Developing one of these types of systems requires the developer to teach the system the specific contextual meanings of the vocabulary.

1.3.6 Availability of natural-language-processing technology

Natural-language-processing technology is less widely available than speech recognition, but there are several commercial systems available that could be integrated with applications. Wit.ai (part of Facebook), Api.ai, and Linguasys are current standalone natural language processing services. OpenNLP, NLULite, NLTK (Loper & Bird 2002), and the Stanford CoreNLP (Stanford University 2014) system are open-source systems that perform linguistic analysis tasks such as part of speech tagging and syntactic analysis. All natural-language-understanding systems have strengths and weaknesses, but for any given application, there will often be one or more suitable system, depending on the application's requirements.

More technical details about speech and natural language processing can be found in Jurafsky and Martin (2008) and Dahl (2013).

1.4 Dialog systems

1.4.1 What are dialog systems?

Dialog systems are systems that interact with the user, understanding what the user says, preparing an appropriate response, and then again listening to the user's response. The system figure (Fig. 1.1), for example, is a full dialog system. Dialog systems include the technologies of speech recognition, natural language understanding, dialog management, natural language generation, and TTS. In this section, we will focus on the technologies for dialog management, which controls the back-and-forth interaction between the system and the user.

Dialog managers vary greatly in their level of sophistication. The simplest form of dialog manager simply reacts to a single user input, independent of context, and produces a simple response, such as text. A more sophisticated dialog manager can take contextual information such as the previous conversation, or even previous interactions with the user, into account and produce complex spoken and graphical responses. Even a simple dialog manager can be very useful, depending on the goals of the application.

In general, a dialog manager will take the output from a natural language understanding system, in the form of a structured meaning, and then decide what the next step in the dialog will be. The next step takes into account not only the structured meaning, but also the purpose and context of the task that the dialog system is trying to accomplish, the user's and the system's previous utterances, aspects of the external context such as the time of day and the location, and the user's and system's previous interactions with each other.

Most dialog systems in common use among the general population are "task oriented". That means they have a task that the system assumes the user is trying to accomplish using the dialog system. This task might be something like making an airline reservation, troubleshooting a faulty product, or describing a medical issue. When the system is developed it will be provided with one or more *task models* that describe the task and the information that has to be obtained from the user before the system can perform the task on the user's behalf. Task-oriented dialogs can be further divided into user-initiative, system-initiative, and mixed-initiative systems. In a user initiative dialog, the user initiates all exchanges. This is sometimes referred to as *command and control*. The system simply passively waits for the user to issue a command, and then it carries it out. This kind of system can be very efficient if the user understands what commands are possible. Unfortunately, this is often not the case, and it can be hard for users to figure out the appropriate commands that can be used to direct the system.

Comparing user initiative to system initiative, in a task like ordering a meal in a restaurant, a user-initiative style utterance might be something like "I would like a roast beef sandwich with onions and lettuce on whole wheat toast, some French fries, and a cup of black coffee", where the user provides all the information about the meal he or she would like to order at once. In a constrained setting like ordering a meal in a restaurant, the user knows what to say because this is a very common situation.

System initiative is a quite different form of interaction where the system asks the user for each piece of information one at a time, and the user is supposed to directly answer each question, without volunteering any extra information, or asking clarifying questions of the system. For example, to order the same meal in a system-initiative system, the interaction might proceed as shown in Fig. 1.15.

System: What filling do you want on your sandwich?
User: roast beef
System: what kind of bread do you want?
User: whole-wheat
System: do you want your bread toasted
User: yes
System: do you want onions on your sandwich?
User: yes
System: do you want tomatoes in your sandwich?
User: no

Fig. 1.15: Food ordering as a directed dialog.

It is clear that this kind of system-directed prompting for each bit of information can be extremely long and tedious for most users and is really only suitable for tasks that are fairly simple with only a few slots to be filled. A good example of a simple system-directed task for the general population might be package tracking where the only slot to be filled is the package tracking number. However, for users with speech and language disabilities who may have difficulty either retrieving the words needed to produce a user-initiative utterance or assembling the ideas into a complete sentence, this form of interaction might be very appropriate.

A more natural type of interaction occurs with the *mixed initiative* type of system. A mixed-initiative system combines prompting by the system with user-initiated questions and information. Normally in a mixed-initiative system, the system will start with a prompt, such as "what kind of sandwich do you want?", which gives the user information about the generally category of responses that the system expects. Knowing then that the system is looking for a description of a sandwich, the user can volunteer the details about the sandwich that they would like to order. If the user does not spontaneously specify all the possible options, then the system can reprompt the user with questions like, "What kind of bread would you like?"

When users have speech or language disorders, the choice between system initiative and user initiative becomes more complex. A heavily system-directed dialog manager may be appropriate for someone with speech or language disorders who has difficulty composing or speaking longer or more complex utterances. In those cases, a short one- or two-word response may be all that the user is capable of. On the other hand, in a remediation context, it may be desirable to encourage the user to produce longer and more complex utterances by increasing the amount of user initiative. This could be done by providing the system with settings that control the amount of system initiative versus user initiative that the system exhibits, with the system either taking its cue from the user's behavior or using a setting supplied by a clinician who is familiar with the user's capabilities.

So far, the discussion has been focused on task-oriented dialogs, where the system and user are collaborating to accomplish a particular task. Not all dialogs are task-oriented. Some dialogs are more socially oriented in that there is no specific goal to be achieved other than to become better acquainted with the other person or share news. In contrast to a task-oriented dialog, an unstructured, non-task-oriented dialog might be something like small talk about the weather or getting general information about such topics as interesting places to visit in a new city. This kind of dialog can also include aspects of a task-oriented dialog; for example, the system might ask the user questions like "what kind of food do you like" or "are you interested in art museums", but

Tab. 1.2: Tasks for different types of dialog systems.

	User initiative	System initiative (directed dialog)	Mixed initiative
Task-oriented	Voice-controlled web browser	Movie schedules, package tracking (simple tasks with few slots)	Food ordering, airline reservations (more complex tasks with many slots), talking to a doctor about medical problems
Unstructured (not task oriented)	Voice web search, chatbot	Discussing interesting places to visit in a new city	Small talk about the weather, social chitchat, talk about your hobbies or family

in general, an unstructured dialog will be less driven toward finding a single correct result for the user than will a task-oriented dialog. Clearly, there is not a distinct dividing line between task- and non-task-oriented dialogs; dialogs can be more or less task-oriented, and the relative task-orientedness can even vary within different stages of the dialog.

Table 1.2 shows examples of tasks that would be appropriate for different dialog styles.

1.4.2 When can dialog systems help?

Task-oriented dialog systems can help users practice specific structured inter-actions, such as ordering food in a restaurant. Commercial telephone dialog systems can be configured so that they listen to a full utterance from the user and accept volunteered information about the task (for example, that the user wants their bread toasted). Then, if required information is missing from the user's utterances, they will prompt the user for the missing information. This mixed-initiative form filling style is supported by the VoiceXML (W3C 2004) dialog standard commonly used in telephone self-help Interactive Voice Res-ponse (IVR) systems. Alternatively, IVRs can also be configured to use a more system-directed style of interaction.

A task-oriented dialog system might be useful in a remediation application for helping users practice specific structured interactions. This would be helpful because it would remove some of the real-time pressure to speak that is inherent in actual dialogs with other people. A system can also be very consistent and regular in its responses. In addition, a system can keep track of many metrics that would be time-consuming for humans to record but could provide a great deal of insight into the user's progress. For example, to quantify the user's progress, the system could keep track of such possible metrics as the following (these metrics are suggested by other work such as the PARADISE model for evaluating spoken dialog systems (Walker, Kamm & Litman 1998) and applications of the EMMA standard discussed in Dahl (2009)):

1. Length of the user's utterances in words (specifically "narrative words" that contribute to the meaning of the utterance, as opposed to corrections, repetitions, or interjections);
2. Number of slots filled with each utterance;
3. Number of slots correctly filled with each utterance;
4. Time between the end of the system's utterance and the beginning of the user's utterance;
5. Well-formedness of the user's utterances;
6. Time required to complete the task;
7. Number of utterances required to complete the task.

A system could also potentially help with traditionally manually coded metrics such as Correct Information Units (Nicholas & Brookshire 1993) and Main Concept Analysis (Nicholas & Brookshire 1995).

Unstructured dialog applications, on the other hand, could be useful by simply allowing users to practice speaking, without having a specific task in mind that they have to accomplish. It might actually reduce stress if the user does not feel like that there is a specific goal that needs to be accomplished in the dialog. Resources for unstructured dialog tasks include the many so-called chatbots that engage in unstructured dialog available on the web, including the original chatbot, ELIZA (see Chatbots (2015) for a list). Metrics in an unstructured dialog application could include some of the same metrics as a structured dialog – specifically latency between utterances and the relative well-formedness of the user's utterances. Although there is no agreed-upon standard for measuring relative well-formedness of an utterance, one metric might be the number of independent fragments required to analyze the sentence as discussed in Norton, Nguyen, Linebarger and Dahl (1993). The strategy discussed in Norton et al. (1993) is based on a parsing strategy where the system attempts to analyze a sentence as if it is fully grammatical. If the sentence is not fully grammatical, the part of the sentence that was parsed up to that point is called a *fragment*, or partial sentence, and the analysis restarts at the point where the failure occurred. This process continues until the end of the sentence is reached. So, if the final analysis contains many fragments, this can be used as a metric that the sentence was not very well-formed.

1.4.3 Limitations of current systems

Although spoken dialog systems are an active area of research, current systems are nevertheless limited in many ways. They are very good at task-oriented slot-filling applications where the slots are relatively independent of each other. They are less successful in more complex situations when the response to one slot affects how subsequent slots are to be understood. For example, a user might ask a system "What time is it in Philadelphia?" followed by "What is the weather like?", meaning "What is the weather like in Philadelphia?". Some systems can go back to the previous utterance to figure out how an utterance should be interpreted, but they usually cannot go much farther back into the conversation than just the previous utterance.

Another limitation of current systems is that they are best at interpreting very literal utterances. For example, if the user said "I hate tomatoes" in response to "Do you want tomatoes on your sandwich?", most systems would be unable to understand that this response should be interpreted as "no, I do not want tomatoes". Similarly, current systems do not handle interruptions very well. For example, if the user were to say, "Excuse me for a second while I get my credit card", very few systems would be able to handle that properly. This is because most systems are developed with a strong focus on talking about and achieving the specific task they are designed to accomplish; it is very unusual for a dialog system to include a baseline set of natural human conversational behaviors. The upshot of these limitations is that interaction with current systems is often not very natural. Although current systems can still be very useful for specific tasks, or for unstructured interactions, many natural conversational behaviors are beyond their capabilities.

Systems that try to fully analyze users' inputs can be good at detecting an ungrammatical input, although they are generally not very good at identifying the exact error. They just know that they failed to find an analysis of the input. If there are only a few possible errors, for example, if the input is very short, users may be able to use this simple form of feedback to revise their inputs and improve their chances of being understood by the system. On the other hand, if the input is long or complex, it can be very difficult and frustrating if the system can only say something like "I did not understand that". Systems that do not try to fully analyze the users' inputs will not be able to provide feedback on well-formedness because they cannot tell the difference between an ungrammatical input and one that is simply off-topic and outside of their domain of expertise.

1.4.4 Availability of dialog system technologies

There are a few current commercial and open-source dialog managers. These include ejTalk (Dahl, Coin, Greene & Mandelbaum 2011), OpenDIAL (open source) (Lison 2013), and AIML (2014). In addition, the W3C's State Chart XML (SCXML) (World Wide Web Consortium 2015) is a standard XML format for state-based applications that can be used to build dialog managers.

Although speech recognition, natural language understanding, and dialog management are the main technologies that are discussed in this book, there are several other speech and language technologies that are worth mentioning briefly.

1.5 Text-to-speech

1.5.1 What is TTS?

Interactive systems often make use of spoken output. Spoken output can be accomplished either with recorded audio files or TTS (a type of *speech synthesis*). Although recorded audio files sound natural and pleasant and are available in any language for which a speaker can be found, they are limited to speaking only outputs that can be anticipated and recorded ahead of time. TTS, on the other hand, can be used to dynamically create text from speech at any point while an application is running.

TTS technology is widely available in desktop computers and mobile devices. In addition, GPS systems often use TTS for eyes-free descriptions of navigation instructions. There is a wide range of quality in TTS systems. For example, most mobile devices and computer operating systems like Windows have very simple TTS systems that are not very pleasant to listen to. This may not be a problem with single words or short sentences, but poor-quality TTS can become very annoying with longer passages.

Although there are some free TTS systems, much-higher-quality TTS technology is available in paid systems. Most TTS systems use some simple forms of natural language processing to perform tasks such as disambiguating homonyms ("lead" the metal versus "lead" the verb, for example). Better-quality TTS systems will also pay attention to punctuation such as commas and question marks, but this is inconsistent from system to system.

Nearly all modern TTS systems are based on a technology called concatenative synthesis, which involves constructing new speech by assembling a sequence of pre-recorded audio snippets or "units" of varying length. When it is time to synthesize the speech, the database of units is searched for units corresponding to the text, and the units are assembled to produce the requested speech. Although concatenative synthesis generally results in the best sounding speech, it is very time-consuming and expensive to develop new voices because thousands of snippets have to be recorded by the speaker the TTS voice will be based on. In addition, the database of speech samples can become very large (generally, the larger the database, the better the speech will sound). The large database can take up large amounts of space on small devices. An earlier technology called formant synthesis generally produces less-pleasant-sounding speech, but its footprint on a device is much smaller and it is easier to develop new voices.

1.5.2 Where could it help?

TTS is widely used by people who are unable to read or who find it very difficult to read printed texts, such as people with impaired vision or dyslexia. TTS is also useful for people who can produce written texts, but who are unable to speak. The physicist Stephen Hawking is a well-known user of TTS, for example.

TTS can also be incorporated into systems to provide audio feedback to users who cannot read or to supplement written feedback. This could help users who need assistance with word retrieval or practice in verbally communicating scripted messages. For example, TTS options in software such as WordQ® (2015) allows the person with aphasia to listen to a written script and then replay it as needed so it serves as a model for repeated verbal practice.

Although TTS can be useful, it does not sound as good as recorded audio, and this raises concerns about the quality and intelligibility of synthesized speech. If feasible (for example, if the feedback consists only of a single word), a more conservative choice would be to use recorded audio (as MossTalk Words does) rather than TTS.

1.5.3 Limits of current systems

Current TTS technology usually has limitations in one of two areas. First, as mentioned above, because most TTS systems are based on concatenative synthesis, transitions between the units are not always completely smooth. As a result, the concatenation process may result in a noticeable audio glitch between segments. This does not usually severely impact intelligibility but it can become a distraction.

The second problem is more apparent in longer stretches of TTS. As a passage of speech being synthesized becomes longer and longer, the changes in intonation, pacing, and emphasis, which reflect the meaning of the text, become more important in ensuring that the speech sounds natural. Because the TTS system does not really understand the text that it is speaking, it is very difficult for it to reproduce these subtle prosodic changes accurately. This is not usually a severe problem, but it does make it hard to listen to long stretches of TTS, especially in texts where prosody plays an important role in the reader's experience, such as fiction. Even if the system pays some attention to punctuation, the prosody will not be nearly as good as that produced by a human reader who actually understands the meaning of the text, because punctuation is only a rough guide to the prosody intended by the author. Certainly, even human readers vary significantly in their ability to read a passage with accurate prosody – good actors will be much more skillful than ordinary readers – so it is not very surprising that TTS still has a long way to go with respect to prosody.

Although fully automatic generation of prosody in TTS systems is quite difficult, there are some manual approaches to improving the quality of prosody in TTS that may be useful.

Speech Synthesis Markup Language (SSML) is an XML notation that can be added to text to describe how the text should be spoken. It is a standard of the World Wide Web Consortium (2012). Fig. 1.16 shows an example of SSML markup for the words "good morning". The meaning of the "contour" attribute (in bold) in the example is that the utterance should start out with the pitch 20 Hz above the baseline; 10% of the way through the utterance, the pitch should rise 30% above the baseline; finally, at 40% of the way into the utterance, the pitch should rise 10 Hz above the baseline. Similarly, SSML provides ways to mark up the text to be synthesized with pauses, speech rate, and volume. Although the format shown in Fig. 1.16 is not very user-friendly, SSML is designed to provide instructions to a TTS system on how to pronounce a particular sentence, so human readability is not very important.

```
<?xml version="1.0"?>
<speak version="1.0" xmlns="http://www.w3.org/2001/10/synthesis"
    xmlns:xsi="http://www.w3.org/2001/XMLSchema-instance"
    xsi:schemaLocation="http://www.w3.org/2001/10/synthesis
        http://www.w3.org/TR/speech-synthesis/synthesis.xsd"
    xml:lang="en-US">
<prosody contour="(0%,+20Hz) (10%,+30%) (40%,+10Hz)">
 good morning
 </prosody>
</speak>
```

Fig. 1.16: SSML example.

There are also tools to aid the process of manually adding SSML markup to text such as Chant VoiceMarkupKit.

Concatenative synthesis is limited in the ability to change the speech rate, because, as mentioned above, concatenative synthesis involves putting together a sequence of audio snippets (called "units") based on actual speech. Changing the rate of speech by a significant amount can introduce unwanted noise into concatenative speech, which can greatly reduce its intelligibility. Formant synthesis, although it does not sound as pleasant as concatenative speech, can be made much faster or slower than the normal rate without adding noise. For this reason, it is often preferred by users of screen readers, who often increase the speech rates of their screen readers in order to listen at very fast rates of speech.

Because the process of creating a high-quality concatenative TTS voice is very time-consuming, the choice of voices is limited. Creating a voice can require 40–50 or more hours of recording time for the person who is doing the recording (normally a professional speaker, sometimes referred to as a "voice talent") to record enough data to produce enough speech so that enough examples of different contexts can be collected. Related to this, good voices will also require significant storage space, so that TTS applications that require local storage of the voice may not be practical on devices with limited storage.

1.5.4 Availability of TTS systems

Developers who wish to incorporate TTS into their own systems have a variety of TTS technologies, of widely varying quality, available to them. Current systems include IVONA, Acapela NeoSpeech, Cepstral, AT&T Natural Voices, Cereproc, and an open-source system from the University of Edinburgh, Festival. In addition to stand-alone TTS systems, complete reading systems are available, such as VoiceDream. Some platforms, such as Android, Apple OSX, or Windows, have a built-in text-speech capability, which can be used by applications, but which is independent of any one application.

Although there are TTS systems available for the several dozen or so most widely spoken languages, there are fewer choices for less common languages.

When people have completely lost the ability to speak or know that they will soon lose the ability to speak, due to a progressive disease or impending surgery, tools are available to create custom voices. A system called ModelTalker has been developed at the University of Delaware to allow people to create a TTS voice based on their own voice or voice of another person of their choosing (Bunnell, Pennington, Yarrington & Gray 2005). VocaliD is a related system that bases new

TTS voices for users who are unable to speak on combinations of the user's voice (if available) and recordings from other people ("donated voices") who match the user as closely as possible in age, gender, dialect, and other parameters that affect voice quality (VocaliD) 2015.

1.6 Natural language generation

1.6.1 What is natural language generation?

Natural language generation is the reverse of natural language understanding; as opposed to extracting structure from a user's natural language utterance, natural language generation starts with a structured representation such as the one in Fig. 1.8 produced by a system, and turns it into language. It is much less widely used than natural language understanding, and full natural language generation, from concepts to language, is still something of a research area. However, for many practical purposes, template-based generation, where different words are inserted into slots in a predefined sentence pattern, is perfectly usable. This is quite common in telephone systems, for example, confirming a pizza order, a system might take a template like, "You have ordered a <size> pizza with <toppings>. Is this correct?" and fill the "size" slot with "large" and fill in the "toppings" slot with "mushrooms and olives" to read back to the user.

More information on natural language generation can be found in Reiter and Dale (2000).

1.6.2 Where could natural language generation help?

Although natural language generation does not seem to have been used in software for speech and language disorders, there are some potential applications. For example, a natural language generation system could take single-word utterances from a user with a limited ability to speak and generate examples of full sentences based on those words. These, in turn, could be presented to the user and the user could select the meaning that they were trying to convey. For example, if the user said "cat ... dog ... chase", the system could offer options like "the cat is chasing the dog", or "the dog is chasing the cat". This would give the user the chance to pick the sentence that best expresses their intention and would give the user some useful feedback on what a more complete version of their utterance would sound like.

1.7 Text simplification

1.7.1 What is text simplification?

Text simplification is a technology for taking a text and changing it so that it is easier to understand. This can involve such techniques as changing the vocabulary, breaking up complex sentences, substituting full noun phrases for pronouns, or defining complex concepts. Although there is a significant body of research literature on the factors that make understanding a text complex (see, for example, Gibson 1998, and the survey in Petersen 2007), work on text simplification technology tends to be based on intuitions about what makes a text difficult to understand more than on psycholinguistic research on human language processing. Sometimes intuitions about complex text are, of course, accurate. Consider this title of an article from the medical journal *Interactive Cardiovascular and Thoracic Surgery* – "Amplatzer occlusion of paravalvular leak of mitral mechanical prosthesis following a reoperation for thrombosed mitral mechanical prosthesis". Clearly, this is hard for most lay people to understand, and looking a little deeper, we can guess that the complexity is largely due to the vocabulary and concepts rather than the syntax. But while intuitions can be useful at times, it would be far better to have actual experimental data on which to base a fuller understanding of the linguistic characteristics of simple or difficult text, and then build these ideas into text simplification software. Evidence for the potential value of text simplification software is the fact that manually simplified text is already being used by people with aphasia (Aphasia Corner 2014).

1.7.2 Where could text simplification help?

In theory, text simplification could be very useful for someone who has difficulty understanding complex language. Software could take a text and create a simpler version that would be easier to read for the user. The user could use a simplified text as an aid to understanding the original text by comparing the simplified text side-by-side with the original text.

1.7.3 Limits of current systems

In practice, text simplification technology is at a very early stage and is not yet very reliable. Also, as mentioned above, the features that are chosen for simplification are often not based on any scientific findings about what makes a text difficult to understand. In addition, existing systems often change the meaning of the text in undesirable ways, or, conversely, do not change the text very much. However, as this technology matures, it is definitely worth keeping in mind for future applications.

1.8 Complementary technologies

Speech and language technologies are often used in conjunction with other related technologies in larger systems. We briefly discuss two of these – artificial intelligence and avatars.

Artificial intelligence refers to a set of technologies that attempt to give computers some of the cognitive abilities of humans. Most of the technologies discussed in this chapter are considered to be subfields of artificial intelligence, especially natural language understanding and dialog management. Other technologies considered to be part of the field of artificial intelligence that which might be useful in applications for people with speech and language disorders are

1. Knowledge representation, used to model facts about the world that a system could talk about;
2. Reasoning, or drawing inferences from sets of facts;
3. Emotion recognition, or identifying emotions from facial expressions, tone of voice, language, or other behaviors;
4. Machine learning, which could be used to automatically learn about user's preferences or skill levels in order to tailor exercises to a particular user.

Fields of artificial intelligence less closely related to this book include object recognition and robotics.

Avatars, or embodied conversational agents, are graphical representations of people or other intelligent agents such as cartoon characters that are used to simulate having a conversation with someone you can see. Avatars can be used to provide a visual representation of a spoken dialog system, or a personality. If the modeling of the facial movements associated with speech is accurate, this visual feedback may help users understand speech output from the avatar. In addition, the presence of a virtual human provides a social presence that make may the user feel more comfortable with the system. On the other hand, a poorly designed avatar will be distracting, confusing, or even unpleasant (Mori 2012). Using avatars as virtual clinicians in aphasia therapy applications has been explored, for example, in Teodoro, Martin, Keshner, Shi and Rudnicky (2013), and is available in the commercial product, AphasiaScripts™ (Rehabilitation Institute of Chicago 2015). Developers who would like to use existing avatar technologies to create their own avatars can look at Make Human™ (2015), an open-source toolkit for making three-dimensional characters. These characters could be integrated into applications for people with language disorders.

1.9 Conclusions

Current speech and language technologies are improving rapidly and are well suited for use in some types of assistive and remediation applications for people with language disorders. Some technical areas, such as speech recognition, TTS, and natural language understanding are fairly mature in terms of technical sophistication, commercial offerings, and development tools. Dialog management and natural language generation are less mature than these technologies; for example, there are very few commercial offerings in these areas. However, they can be used (especially in a simplified form) in many applications. Other technologies, such as text simplification and prosodic analysis, are less mature and are likely to be available primarily in research systems. The range of variation in maturity of speech and language technologies means that incorporation of the technologies into systems for people with speech and language disorders must be considered carefully in the context of the specific goals of the application, recognizing that even the most mature technologies will make occasional errors. As a consequence, error handling will always be an importance consideration in these systems.

References

AIML 2.0 working draft. (2014). Retrieved February 3, 2015. http://www.alicebot.org/aiml.html

Aphasia Corner. (2014). *Newsela: Leveling reading difficulty.* Retrieved March 28, 2015, from http://aphasiacorner.com/blog/uncategorized/newsela-leveling-reading-difficulty-1541

Bunnell, H. T., Pennington, C., Yarrington, D. & Gray, J. (2005). Automatic personal synthetic voice construction. In *Eurospeech 2005*, Lisbon, Portugal.

Chatbots. (2015). *Virtual agents/Chatbots directory.* at https://www.chatbots.org/

Dahl, D. A. (2009). *Improving dialogs with EMMA. SpeechTEK.* New York: Information Today, Inc.

Dahl, D. A. (2013). Natural language processing: Past, present and future. In: A. Neustein & J. Markowitz (Eds.), *Mobile speech and advanced natural language solutions.* Springer, New York, NY, USA.

Dahl, D. A., Coin, E., Greene, M. & Mandelbaum, P. (2011). A conversational personal assistant for senior users. In D. Perez-Marin & I. Pascual-Nieto (Eds.), *Conversational agents and natural language interaction: Techniques and effective practices.* Hershey, PA: IGI Global, 282–301.

Gibson, E. (1998). Linguistic complexity: Locality of syntactic dependencies. *Cognition, 68*, 1–76.

Jurafsky, D. & Martin, J. (2008). *Speech and language processing: An introduction to natural language processing*, 2nd ed. Prentice-Hall, Upper Saddle River, New Jersey.

Kartal, G. (2006). Working with an imperfect medium: Speech recognition technology in reading practice. *Journal of Educational Multimedia and Hypermedia, 15(3)*, 303–328.

Lee, K.-F. (1989). *Automatic speech recognition: The development of the SPHINX system.* Norwell, MA: Kluwer Academic Publishers.

Lison, P. (2013). *Structured probabilistic modelling for dialogue management.* PhD thesis, University of Oslo, Oslo, Norway.

Loper, E. & Bird, S. (2002). NLTK: The Natural Language Toolkit. In *ACL Workshop on Effective Tools and Methodologies for Teaching Natural Language Processing and Computational Linguistics, 40th Annual Meeting of the Association for Computational Linguistics*, July 11–12, 2002, Philadelphia, PA.

Make Human™. (2015). *MakeHuman open source tool for making 3D characters.* Retrieved March 18, 2015, from http://www.makehuman.org/

Mori, M. (2012). The uncanny valley. *IEEE Robotics & Automation Magazine*, 98–100.

Nicholas, L. E. & Brookshire, R. H. (1993). A system for scoring main concepts in the discourse of non-brain damaged and aphasic speakers. *Clinical Aphasiology, 21*, 87–99.

Nicholas, L. E. & Brookshire, R. H. (1995). Presence, completeness, and accuracy of main concepts in the connected speech of non-brain-damaged adults and adults with aphasia. *Journal of speech and Hearing Research, 38*, 145–153.

Norton, L. M., Nguyen, N., Linebarger, M. C. & Dahl, D. A. (1993). Integrating speech recognition and natural language understanding to process air traffic control instructions. In *3rd Annual 1993 IEEE Mohawk Valley Section Dual-Use Technologies and Applications Conference*, 1993 May 24–27, Rome, NY, pp. 102–107.

Panttaja, E. M. (1988). *Recognizing intonational patterns in English speech.* BS thesis, Massachusetts Institute of Technology, Cambridge, MA.

Petersen, S. E. (2007). Natural language processing tools for reading level assessment and text simplification for bilingual education [PhD thesis]: University of Washington.

Rehabilitation Institute of Chicago. (2015). *AphasiaScripts™.* Retrieved March 18, 2015, from http://ricaphasiascripts.contentshelf.com/welcome

Reiter, E. & Dale, R. (2000). *Building natural language generation systems.* Cambridge, UK: Cambridge University Press.

Scientific Learning. (2015). *Reading Assistant™.* Retrieved March 18, 2015, from http://www.scilearn.com/

Shivakumar, P., Potamianos, A., Lee, S. & Narayanan, S. (2014, September). Improving speech recognition for children using acoustic adaptation and pronunciation modeling. In *Proceedings of Workshop on Child Computer Interaction (WOCCI 2014)*, Singapore.

Stanford University. (2014). *Stanford CoreNLP.* Retrieved from http://nlp.stanford.edu/software/corenlp.shtml

Teodoro, G., Martin, N., Keshner, E., Shi, J. Y. & Rudnicky, A. I. (2013). Virtual clinicians for the treatment of aphasia and speech disorders. *Virtual rehabilitation (IVVR)* (pp. 158–159). Philadelphia, PA: IEEE.

The CMU Sphinx Group. (2009). *The CMU Sphinx Group open source speech recognition engines.* Retrieved January 16, 2015, from http://cmusphinx.sourceforge.net/html/cmusphinx.php

Vicsi, K. & Szaszák, G. (2010). Using prosody to improve automatic speech recognition. *Speech Communication, 52,* 413–426.

VocaliD. VocaliD, (2015). (Accessed March 4, 2015, at https://www.vocalid.co/.)

W3C. (2004). *Voice Extensible Markup Language (VoiceXML 2.0).* Retrieved November 9, 2012, from http://www.w3.org/TR/voicexml20/

W3C. (2004). *W3C speech recognition grammar specification (SRGS).* Retrieved November 9, 2012, from http://www.w3.org/TR/speech-grammar/

Walker, M., Kamm, C. & Litman, D. (1998). Toward developing general models of usability with PARADISE. *Natural Language Engineering, 6,* 363–377.

Williams, S. M., Nix, D. & Fairweather, P. (2000). Using speech recognition technology to enhance literacy instruction for emerging readers. In B. Fishman & S. O'Connor-Divelbiss (Eds.), *Fourth International Conference of the Learning Sciences* (pp. 115–120). Mahwah, NJ: Erlbaum.

WordQ. (2015). *WordQ.* Retrieved from http://www.synapseadaptive.com/quillsoft/WQ/wordq_features.htm

World Wide Web Consortium. (2012). *State Chart XML (SCXML): State machine notation for control abstraction.* Retrieved November 20, 2012, from http://www.w3.org/TR/scxml/

Katharine Beals
2 Overview of developmental language disorders

Abstract: This chapter describes the developmental language disorders that are the focus of the next three chapters: dyslexia, Specific Language Impairment (SLI), and autism spectrum disorders.

Developmental language disorders are language disorders that emerge in the course of childhood. At their core are impairments in the processing of linguistic information, whether of speech sounds, grammar (syntax and/or morphology), semantics (meaning), and/or pragmatics (language use). These impairments may affect language comprehension (receptive language), language production (expressive language), or both.

The major developmental language impairments, or impairments that include language impairment, are phonological processing disorders, specific language impairment (SLI), and autism spectrum disorders. One set of developmental disorders that we do not address here are those that are specific to speech production, or the oral articulation of language: the movements of tongue, lips, and other parts of the speech apparatus that produce speech sounds. Speech-specific disorders involve mechanisms like motor coordination and planning that are not generally considered specific to, or central to language, or to the capacity to learn language.

We also will not focus on general cognitive delays, as these are grounded in more general learning and information processing skills. However, since cognitive delays can delay language learning and language processing, affected children may have what we call here a "general language impairment", and some of what we discuss in terms of remediation needs will apply to this population.

The same goes for children with hearing impairments/deafness and auditory processing impairments. The latter, it should be noted, is a controversial diagnostic category whose clinical validity has been disputed. Hearing impairments affect perception and discrimination of sound in general rather than speech sounds in particular – and the same is said to be true of auditory processing disorders. But since speech comprises the most complex sounds we process, and since both hearing impairments and auditory processing impairments can distort sound perception and delay language acquisition, some of what we discuss here in terms of remediation needs will also apply to children with hearing impairments, deafness, and/or auditory processing impairments. This is especially true of partial hearing impairment, as it often selectively affects high frequency sounds that include those of consonants and, in particular, the consonantal word endings that mark past tense ("walked"), third person singular simple present ("he/she walks"), and plurals ("cups", "beds").

Returning now to the language-specific deficits that are our focus, let us begin with phonological processing impairments. Phonological processing involves the discrimination and processing of the smallest distinctive sounds that make up language, otherwise known as phonemes (and generally classified as consonants or vowels). The major disorder associated with phonological processing is dyslexia, although some have observed phonological processing deficits in subsets of children with autism and SLI (see Rapin & Dunn 2003; Tallal & Fitch 2004). The latest research on dyslexia actually suggests two underlying deficits: a delay in the ability to rapidly name objects (which involves impairment in automatic retrieval from long-term memory) and a diminished awareness of phonemes (the basis for the phonological processing impairment) (see Wolf 2007). Diminished phonemic awareness can subtly impair speech perception, potentially resulting in delays in language acquisition (Joanisse, Manis, Keating & Seidenberg 2000). But the most obvious problems are in areas that require conscious phonological awareness: namely, breaking words down into phonemes and building words up from phonemes. In the many writing systems that, like English (for all its irregularities), are based mostly on phonemes, an essential subskill of reading is the decoding of written words. Thus, although dyslexia is essentially a language disorder, it most obviously affects reading. And, even though its most direct effect on reading is to impair the decoding of written words, it can create a bottleneck in the acquisition of reading skills, and in the reading process itself, that, in turn, can impede higher-level reading comprehension. Dyslexia may also cause difficulties with spelling, as spelling depends, in part, on the ability to break words down into phonemes.

Another disorder that is specifically grounded in language, as its name suggests, is Specific Language Impairment (SLI). SLI is a somewhat heterogeneous category diagnosed on the basis of language levels that, in the absence of other conditions like hearing loss, autism, or general cognitive impairment, fall significantly below age level. Typically, people with SLI have non-verbal IQ scores in the normal range, but their performance on tests of vocabulary or grammatical ability fall more than one standard deviation below the mean. Some children with dyslexia diagnoses, it should be noted, also meet these criteria.

Some studies (Kjelgaard & Tager-Flusberg 2001) have found grammar in SLI to be more impaired than vocabulary, and grammar limitations in productive language to be particularly salient (Leonard 1998). In terms of productive grammar, people with SLI have difficulty using proper verb morphology (Bishop 1994; Clahsen, Bartke & Göllner 1997; van der Lely, Heather & Ullman 2001) and certain syntactic structures like passives (van der Lely 1996; Norbury, Bishop & Briscoe 2001) and wh-questions (van der Lely & Battell 2003). Also challenging is verb argument structure – that is, combining verbs with appropriate direct and indirect objects ("arguments"). For example, some studies have found SLI children, even those older than 7 years, to omit obligatory arguments – e.g. the indirect object "me" in "Give me a book" (Thordardottir & Ellis Weismer 2002). With so-called change-of-state verbs like "fill" and "cover", they also produce such errors as "The lady is filling the sweets into the jar" and "The lady is covering the scarf on her head" (Ebbels, Dockrell & van der Lely 2012; Ebbels, van der Lely & Dockrell 2007).

Receptive grammar, or comprehension of grammatical meaning, is also affected, with SLI children having difficulty understanding grammatically complex constructions (Bishop 1979, 1982; Bishop & Adams 1990; van der Lely & Harris 1990; Montgomery 1995; van der Lely & Stollwerck 1997) and judging sentences for grammaticality (Rice, Wexler & Redmond 1999). Some (Rapin & Allen 1983, 1987) have proposed that in addition to a grammar-impaired group within SLI, there is also a subgroup whose relative deficits are in comprehension. Comprehension impairments, it is worth noting, have also been implicated in attention deficit disorders (see, for example, Purvis 1997), and such impairments ultimately affect not just spoken language, but written language as well.

Returning to grammar difficulties in particular, SLI and a grammar-impaired subgroup of children with autism have been found to have both genetic and linguistic overlap, particularly in the area of grammatical morphology, for example, in past tense marking ("walked") and third person singular simple present ("he/she walks") (Kjelgaard & Tager-Flusberg 2001; Roberts, Rice & Tager-Flusberg 2004).

Turning to autism spectrum disorders more generally, autism, unlike dyslexia and SLI, is not, first and foremost, a language-specific disorder. Across the entire autism spectrum, from low functioning to high functioning, just one aspect of language is universally impaired: pragmatics, particularly the social aspects of language use. Given that deficits in social awareness and social reciprocity are among the core deficits in autism, this is hardly surprising. But pragmatic deficits, even on their own, can be highly debilitating, hindering functional communication even in those with superior vocabulary skills (Marans, Rubin & Laurent 2005; Lewis, Murdoch & Woodyatt 2007). One specific pragmatic difficulty exhibited by many children with autism is the distinction among first, second, and third person pronouns ("I"/"me"; "you"; "he"/"she") (see Szatmari, Bartolucci & Bremner 1989). In the past, individuals whose only linguistic deficits were in pragmatics were diagnosed with Asperger syndrome, or alternatively, with semantic-pragmatic disorder. Asperger syndrome no longer appears in the *Diagnostic and Statistical Manual of Mental Disorders*; in its place is Social (Pragmatic) Communication Disorder. Because so much of what is communicated requires pragmatic reasoning for full comprehension, deficits in pragmatics, even unaccompanied by other linguistic deficits, are associated with deficits in language comprehension in general and in reading comprehension in particular.

Although pragmatics is the only aspect of language that is universally impaired in autism, many individuals with moderate to severe autism experience impediments and/or delays in all aspects of language, and this is partly, if not wholly, due to factors that are specific to autism. Neuropsychological evidence suggests that those with autism have reduced orienting responses and attention to speech sounds (Ceponiene et al. 2003) – responses that, in typical children, facilitate first-language acquisition (Kuhl, Coffey-Corina, Padden & Dawson 2005). Additional deficits in joint attention and social interest cause children with autism to miss opportunities to map linguistic input to a speaker's intentions – a crucial bootstrapping mechanism in typical language acquisition (Baldwin & Moses 1996; Happe & Loth 2002). In particular, joint attention deficits substantially impede the acquisition of word meanings (see Bloom 2002).

As it turns out, however, at least among the majority on the spectrum who do have verbal skills, the greatest deficits in autism are not in vocabulary. Vocabulary, indeed, tends to be a relative strength, so much so as to cause overestimates of overall linguistic competence (Tager-Flusberg 1988; Mottron 2007). Far greater, relatively speaking, are deficits, not just in pragmatics, but also in grammar. Even when vocabulary acquisition is age appropriate, individuals with autism can exhibit syntactic errors (Kjelgaard & Tager-Flusberg 2001; Roberts et al. 2004; Kelley, Paul, Fein & Naigles 2006). One study estimates that about one third of the population with autism present with signs of a comorbid language impairment that specifically affects grammar (Kjelgaard & Tager-Flusberg 2001, but also see Whitehouse & Bishop 2008). Others find that phonological and syntactic deficits characterize 65% of the population, contradicting the once common belief that verbal individuals with autism are relatively unimpaired in these areas (Rapin & Dunn 2003). Generally, children with autism are more likely to make syntactic and morphosyntactic errors, and they tend to speak in shorter, less complex utterances than control subjects matched on vocabulary acquisition and non-verbal mental age (Tager-Flusberg et al. 1997; Eigsti, Bennetto & Dadlani 2007; Eigsti, Marchena, Schuh & Kelley 2011). Even in the absence of a specific language impairment, the social and attentional characteristics of autism can still cause syntactic or pragmatic language delays (Minshew, Goldstein & Siegel 1995). These, in turn, affect productive language, receptive language, and reading comprehension.

In all three disorders, linguistic competence is highly correlated with achievement and long-term outcome; this is particularly true of autism (Garfin & Lord 1986; Committee on Educational Interventions for Children with Autism 2001; Prizant & Whetherby 2005). Given that most instruction is mediated through language, whether by teachers or by textbooks, receptive language impairments are especially debilitating. For example, among individuals with SLI, those whose receptive language impairments persist into school have a particularly poor prognosis (Stothard, Snowling, Bishop, Chipchase & Kaplan 1998; Mawhood, Howlin & Rutter 2000). In the later grades, when students move from learning to read to reading to learn, deficits in reading comprehension in particular – with which, as we discussed, all of these disorders are associated – become ever more academically debilitating.

It is notable that all three types of language impairment are characterized by something specific that interferes with normal language acquisition, whether it is an under-awareness of phonemes in dyslexia, an under-awareness of grammatical forms in SLI, or an under-awareness of social interactions and a diminished orientation to human voices in autism. In a way, all three populations resemble second-language learners, each one needing more simplified and/or systematic exposure to language than real life provides. These children, then, may be particularly suited to systematic remediation programs of the sort that computerized technologies are poised to provide. The first step in this process is a thorough assessment of linguistic skills and deficits: the opening topic of Chapter 3.

References

Baldwin, D. & Moses, L. (1996). The ontogeny of social information gathering. *Child Development, 67*, 1915–1939.

Bishop, D. V. M. (1979). Comprehension in developmental language disorders. *Developmental Medicine and Child Neurology, 21*, 225–238.

Bishop, D. V. M. (1982). Comprehension of spoken, written, and signed sentences in childhood language disorders. *Journal of Child Psychology and Psychiatry, 23*, 20.

Bishop, D. V. M. (1994). Grammatical errors in specific language impairment: Competence or performance limitation? *Applied Psycholinguistics*, 15.

Bishop, D. V. M. & Adams, C. (1990). A prospective study of the relationship between specific language impairment, phonological disorders and reading retardation. *Journal of Child Psychology and Psychiatry, 31*, 1027–1050.

Bloom, P. (2002). Mindreading, communication, and learning the names for things. *Mind & Language, 17*, 37–54.

Ceponiene, R., Lepistö, T., Shestakova, A., Vanhala, R., Näätänen, R. & Yaguchi, K. (2003). Speech sound-selective auditory impairment in infantile autism: Can perceive but will not attend. *Proceedings of the National Academy of Sciences of the United States of America, 100*, 5567–5572.

Clahsen, H., Bartke, S. & Göllner, S. (1997). Formal features in impaired grammars: A comparison of English and German children. *Journal of Neurolinguistics, 10*, 151–171.

Committee on Educational Interventions for Children with Autism. (2001). Educating Children with Autism. In Education DoBaSSa (Ed.). Washington, DC: National Academy Press.

Ebbels, S. H., Dockrell, J. E. & van der Lely, H. K. (2012). Production of change-of-state, change-of-location and alternating verbs: A comparison of children with specific language impairment and typically developing children. *Language and Cognitive Processes, 27*, 1312–1333.

Ebbels, S. H., van der Lely, H. K. & Dockrell, J. E. (2007). Intervention for verb argument structure in children with persistent SLI: A randomized control trial. *Journal of Speech Language and Hearing Research, 50*, 1330–1349.

Eigsti, I., Bennetto, L. & Dadlani, M. (2007). Beyond pragmatics: Morphosyntactic development in autism. *Journal of Autism Development and Disorder, 37*, 1007–1023.

Eigsti, I., Marchena, A. B., Schuh, J. M. & Kelley, E. (2011). Language acquisition in autism spectrum disorders: A developmental review. *Research in Autism Spectrum Disorders, 5*, 681–691.

Garfin, D. G. & Lord, C. (1986). *Communication as a social problem in autism*. New York: Plenum Press.

Happe, F. & Loth, E. (2002). 'Theory of mind' and tracking speakers' intentions. *Mind & Language, 17*, 24–36.

Joanisse, M. F., Manis, F. R., Keating, P. & Seidenberg, M. S. (2000). Language deficits in dyslexic children: Speech perception, phonology, and morphology. *Journal of Experimental Child Psychology, 77*, 30–60.

Kelley, E., Paul, J. P., Fein, D. & Naigles, L. (2006). Residual language deficits in optimal outcome children with a history of autism. *Journal of Autism Development and Disorder, 36*, 807–828.

Kjelgaard, M. M. & Tager-Flusberg, H. (2001). An investigation of language impairment in autism: Implications for genetic subgroups. *Language and Cognitive Processes, 16*, 287–308.

Kuhl, P. K., Coffey-Corina, S., Padden, D. & Dawson, D. (2005). Links between social and linguistic processing of speech in preschool children with autism: Behavioral and electrophysiological measures. *Developmental Science, 8*.

Leonard, L. B. (1998). *Children with specific language impairment*. Cambridge, MA: MIT Press.

Lewis, F. M., Murdoch, B. E. & Woodyatt, G. C. (2007). Communicative competence and metalinguistic ability: Performance by children and adults with autism spectrum disorder. *Journal of Autism and Developmental Disorders, 38*, 1525–1538.

Marans, W. D., Rubin, E. & Laurent, A. (2005). Addressing social communication skills in individuals with high functioning autism and Asperger syndrome: critical priorities in educational programming. In F. R. Volkmar, A. Klin & R. Paul (Eds.), *Handbook of autism and pervasive developmental disorders*, 3rd ed. (pp. 977–1002). New York: John Wiley.

Mawhood, L., Howlin, P. & Rutter, M. (2000). Autism and developmental receptive language disorder – a comparative follow-up in early adult life: I. Cognitive and language outcomes *Journal of Child Psychology and Psychiatry, 41*, 547–559.

Minshew, N. J., Goldstein, G. & Siegel, D. J. (1995). Speech and language in high functioning autistic individuals. *Neuropschology, 9*, 255–261.

Montgomery, J. W. (1995). Sentence comprehension in children with specific language impairment: The role of phonological working memory. *Journal of Speech and Hearing Research, 38*.

Mottron, L. (2007). Matching strategies in cognitive research with individuals with high-functioning autism: Current practices, instrument biases, and recommendations. *Journal of Autism Development and Disorder, 34*, 19–27.

Norbury, C. F., Bishop, D. V. M. & Briscoe, J. (2001). Production of English finite verb morphology: A comparison of SLI and mild-moderate hearing impairment. *Journal of Speech, Language and Hearing Research, 44*, 165–178.

Prizant, B. M. & Whetherby, A. M. (2005). Enhancing communication abilities for person with autism spectrum disorders. In F. Volkmar, R. Paul, A. Klin & D. Cohen (Eds.), *Handbook of autism and pervasive developmental disorders* (pp. 929–945). Hoboken, NJ: Wiley & Sons.

Purvis, K. L, T. R. (1997). Language abilities in children with attention deficit hyperactivity disorder, reading disabilities, and normal controls. *Journal of Abnormal Child Psychology,* 133–144.

Rapin, I. & Allen, D. (1983). Developmental language disorders: Nosologic considerations. In U. Kirk (Ed.), *Neuropsychology of language, reading, and spelling* (pp. 155–184). New York: Academic Press.

Rapin, I. & Allen, D. (1987). Developmental dysphasia and autism in preschool children: Characteristics and subtypes. In J. Martin, P. Fletcher, P. Grunwell & D. Hall (Eds.), *Proceedings of the First International Symposium on Specific Speech and Language Disorders in Children* (pp. 20–35). London: Afasic.

Rapin, I. & Dunn, M. (2003). Update on the language disorders of individuals on the autistic spectrum. *Brain & Development, 25*, 166–172.

Rice, M. L., Wexler, K. & Redmond, S. M. (1999). Grammaticality judgments of an extended optional infinitive grammar: Evidence from English-speaking children with specific language impairment. *Language and Hearing Research, 42*, 943–961.

Roberts, J. A., Rice, M. L. & Tager-Flusberg, H. (2004). Tense marking in children with autism. *Applied Psycholinguistics, 25*, 429–448.

Stothard, S. E., Snowling, M. J., Bishop, D. V. M., Chipchase, B. B. & Kaplan, C. A. (1998). Language impaired preschoolers: a follow-up into adolescence. *Journal of Speech, Language and Hearing Research, 41*, 407–418.

Szatmari, P., Bartolucci, G. & Bremner, R. (1989). Asperger's syndrom and autism: Comparison of early history and outcome. *Developmental Medicin and CHild Neurology, 31*, 709–720.

Tager-Flusberg, H. (1988). On the nature of a language acquisition disorder: The example of autism. In F. Kessel (Ed.), *Development of language and language researchers: Essays in honor of Roger Brown* (pp. 249–267). Hillsdale, NJ: Lawrence Earlbaum.

Tager-Flusberg, H., Lord, C. & Paul, R. (1997). Language and communication in autism. In D. J. Cohen & F. R. Volkmar (Eds.), *Handbook of autism and pervasive developmental disorders* (pp. 195–225). New York: John Wiley & Sons.

Tallal, P. & Fitch, H. (2004). Central auditory processing and language learning impairments: Implications for neuroplasticity research. In J. Syka & M. M. Merzenich (Eds.), *Plasticity and signal representation in the auditory system* (pp. 355–385). New York: Kluwer Plenum.

Thordardottir, E. T. & Ellis Weismer, S. (2002). Verb argument structure weakness in SLI in relation to age and utterance length. *Clinical Linguistics and Phonetics, 16*, 233–250.

van der Lely, H. K. (1996). Specifically language impaired and normally developing children: Verbal passive vs adjectival passive sentence interpretation. *Lingua, 98*, 243–272.

van der Lely, H. K. & Battell, J. (2003). Wh-movement in children with grammatical SLI: A test of the RDDR hypothesis. *Language, 79*, 153–181.

van der Lely, H. K. & Harris, M. (1990). Comprehension of reversible sentences in specifically language impaired children. *Journal of Speech and Hearing Disorders, 55*, 101–117.

van der Lely, H. K. & Stollwerck, L. (1997). Binding theory and specifically language impaired children. *Cognition, 62*, 245–290.

van der Lely, H. K. J., Heather, K. J. & Ullman, M. T. (2001). Past tense morphology in specifically language impaired and normally developing children. *Language and Cognitive Processes, 16*, 177–217.

Whitehouse, A. J. O. & Bishop, D. V. M. (2008). Do children with autism 'switch off' to speech sounds? An investigation using event-related potentials. *Developmental Science, 11*, 516–524.

Wolf, M. (2007). Proust and the squid: The story and science of the reading brain. Harper Collins, New York: NY.

Katharine Beals
3 Technology for assessment and remediation of developmental language disorders

Abstract: This chapter discusses potential and existing technologies for assessing and remediating developmental language disorders. The first section discusses how technology can supplement traditional in-person assessments. The next section discusses how technology can supplement traditional remediations. Two subsections follow: first, a review of technologies that address receptive language; next, a review of technologies that address productive language. This last subsection focuses, in particular, on the GrammarTrainer, a software program created by the author of this chapter.

The specific developmental language disorders we are focusing on, once again, are phonological processing disorders, specific language impairment (SLI), and autism (see Chapter 2 for discussion). Therefore, the technologies that we discuss here are those that address language in general, as opposed to speech in particular.

3.1 Linguistic technologies for assessing language needs

One of the first steps in addressing the needs of those with developmental language disorders is determining what sort of remediation is necessary and placing the student appropriately within a remediation program. In this section, we explore ways in which linguistic technologies can complement existing assessment tools.

Traditional assessments are well suited to certain aspects of language. One area is vocabulary. Vocabulary tests are also easily computerized – substantially sparing the manpower of traditional assessments. But vocabulary by itself gives an incomplete picture of language skills, especially given that, in both autism and SLI, it tends to be a relative strength compared with grammar and (in the case of autism) pragmatics.

Traditional in-person assessments, as well as surveys of parents and teachers – seen for example in the pragmatics section of the commonly used Clinical Evaluation of Language Fundamentals (CELF) test – can also give a good sense of a child's overall pragmatics skills. In contrast to vocabulary assessments, pragmatics assessments are not well suited to computerization. First, it is difficult for computers to simulate the real-world contexts in which day-to-day pragmatics plays out: school yards, classrooms, cafeterias, group discussions, etc. Second, the vast range of possible pragmatically appropriate responses to any given situation or simulation makes it difficult for a program to assess whether a given response is pragmatically felicitous. Consider, for example, "Who is she?", uttered in response to "I'm leaving": depending on the situation, it might be a total non-sequitur, or it might be the perfect retort.

Traditional assessments, for example, the Understanding Spoken Paragraphs section of the CELF test, are also well suited to assessing discourse and text-level comprehension. Given the open-endedness of some of the reading comprehension questions – "What is this story about?" and "Why do you think Ying was putting her socks on slowly?", to take two sample questions from the CELF – the user's responses are again much better evaluated face-to-face by humans than automatically by computers.

When it comes to grammar, however, traditional assessments only go so far. Although the available speech therapist-delivered grammar assessments are fairly broad and linguistically informed, they overlook many of the more advanced grammar skills. This is true both of receptive grammar assessments and of productive grammar assessments.

Before examining these assessments, let us clarify the terms "receptive grammar" and "productive grammar". Receptive grammar, as with receptive language in general, is about comprehension – in this case, the comprehension of grammatical structures. Similarly, as with productive language, productive grammar is about producing – producing grammatical structures. Generally, in the course of language development, receptive grammar – like receptive language – develops ahead of productive grammar: comprehension precedes production. Production, moreover, requires active recall, while reception can rely more on passive recognition. As we have seen, both receptive and productive language can be impaired in children with developmental language delays.

In terms of receptive grammar, the standard human-administered measures are the Sentence Comprehension, Linguistics Concepts, and Following Directions components of the CELF test, as well as Dorothy Bishop's Test of Receptive Grammar (TROG). All involve the examiner prompting the child with a series of oral sentence prompts, accompanying each prompt with a picture or set of pictures. The child selects the picture, or the element in the picture, that goes with the prompt. The sentence prompts range in complexity from basic sentences like "Point to the circle" and "The girl lost her balloon" to more complex ones that include passives ("The girl is being pushed by the boy"), as well as negated sentences ("The cow is not running"), sentences with coordinate structures ("Point to the white circle and the black square"; "The boy is chasing the dog and is jumping"; "The box is neither big nor yellow"), sentences with comparative structures ("The tree is taller than the house"), and sentences containing relative clauses in various positions of the sentence ("The book that is red is on the pencil"; "The man pushes the cow that is standing"; "The man the elephant sees is sitting"). These tests also assess comprehension of third person pronouns ("She is pointing at them"; "The boy sees that the elephant is touching him").

The downside of tests that only measure receptive grammar, or comprehension, is that they do not give a complete picture of a child's grammar skills. Consider, for example, negated sentences like "The cow is not running" or "The cow did not run". Comprehending such sentences is different from actively constructing them. In the first case, one simply recognizes the presence of a negating element (e.g. "not"). In the second case, one has to go through the process of placing the negative after the auxiliary verb (e.g. "is"), or, if there is no auxiliary, inserting the appropriate form of the auxiliary verb "do" (e.g. "did"). The same goes for passively recognizing vs. actively constructing a question (see Section 3.2). While a child may have learned to attend to particular linguistic elements (e.g. to search for the -s ending to determine plurality), the capacity to produce a given construction may require practice actually producing it (Clahsen & Felser 2006). Preliminary data by Hurewitz and Beals (2008) (see Section 3.2 for details) find students generally performing worse when asked to produce correct grammatical structures than when asked merely to identify them. In short, receptive measures of grammar are incomplete measures of grammar skills and should be accompanied by productive measures – as they are in the CELF test.

The standard tests of productive grammar – or of the range of grammatical structures that a child is able to produce – are the Word Structure, Formulated Sentences, and Sentence Assembly components of the CELF test, the Syntax Construction subtest of the Comprehensive Assessment of Spoken Language (CASL), the South Tyneside Assessment of Syntactic Structures (the STASS), and the Index of Productive Syntax (or IPSyn, see Scarborough 1990). The IPSyn is unique among these in that it is designed for preschool-aged children and in that, rather than testing a child on particular grammatical structures, it samples the child's spontaneous speech, elicited via an examiner who has him or her retell stories and answer various questions. After a child's speech is recorded, 100 of his or her utterances are transcribed and analyzed for particular grammatical features and structures (noun phrases, verb phrases, questions, negations, and various basic sentence structures). Given that the more complex structures that distinguish the speech of more linguistically advanced children are relatively less likely to show up in this sort of relatively small language sample, the IPSyn is most appropriate for assessing basic grammar skills.

The CELF, STASS, and CASL probe more advanced skills, deploying a more constrained testing environment that returns us to the oral-prompt-plus-picture format seen above with the receptive grammar tests. But here the examiner, rather than having the child point to a picture, uses a picture plus an oral prompt to get the child to produce a specific syntactic structure. For example, in the CELF's Word Structure section, the child hears prompts like "This boy is (point) standing and this boy is ... (point)", with the examiner pointing first to a picture of a boy standing and then to one of a boy sitting, and where the target is "sitting". This particular section tests regular plural, irregular plural, possessive nouns, third person singular verb forms ("she swims"), regular and irregular past tense, future tense, present progressive, pronoun forms, and auxiliaries. The STASS test and the Formulated Sentences part of the CELF test are more open-ended: the picture may be fairly complicated, and the guiding prompt may consist of a single, spoken word. For example, in a practice exercise of the Formulated Sentences subtest, the examiner asks the child to use the word "when" to describe a cafeteria scene with children sitting at a table, a child ordering food, and another child throwing out the contents of a tray.

The Sentence Assembly component of the CELF test uses a different tactic to elicit syntactic formations, presenting the child with a list of scrambled words and phrases and prompting him or her to unscramble them to form two different sentences. Examples range from lists like (1) "tall", "the boy", "is", (answer: "The boy is tall" and "Is the boy tall?") and (2) "saw", "the girl", "the boy", to considerably more complex lists like (3) "the runner", "the race", "to win", "going", "is not" and (4) "the keys", "the girl", "her pocket", "put", "did not", "in". In all, it has the student constructing a variety of different declarative and interrogative sentences, including ones involving passive voice, negation, infinitive phrases, and relative and other subordinate clauses.

These productive grammar tests, while tapping into aspects of active grammar knowledge that the receptive tests neglect, still have their limitations. In the case of the IPSyn, the limitation is what the child happens to generate in the way of spontaneous speech. Those 100 sampled utterances may or may not include a representative set of grammatical structures. In one study of the IPSyn in particular (Hewitt, Hammer, Yont & Tomblin 2005), especial difficulty was found in eliciting questions: the children seemed to expect the examiner to be the one asking the questions, and were not comfortable asking questions themselves; many of the language samples contained two or fewer questions.

In the case of the CELF, STASS, and CASL, the limitations pertain instead to which structures can be elicited from the child without giving too much away. Consider, for example, passive voice. How do you prompt a child to use the passive form of a sentence rather than its active counterpart in describing a particular picture – say of a dog biting a man? How do you get the child to say "The man was bitten by the dog?" rather than "The dog bit the man"? You might ask the child to start with the word "man", but what do you do if the child says, "The man is hurt"? You might tell the child to use the word "bite", but then the child might say, "The man was hurt after the dog bit him". Other forms are even more difficult to elicit. It is easy to prompt the child to answer a wh-question, but how do you prompt him to ask one? The more open-ended parts of these tests run into a problem similar to that of the IPSyn: the child may or may not produce anything close to the hoped-for structure, even if he or she has it in his or her grammatical repertoire. For example, returning to the "when" prompt and the complicated cafeteria scene, a child might say anything from "When is lunch over?" to "When the kids finish eating, they throw out their trays".

Because it tells students exactly which words and phrases to use, the Sentence Assembly word-unscrambling strategy gets further with elicitation, but only at the expense of giving away clues. For example, part of what's challenging about the passive voice is using the past participle form of the verb (e.g. "bitten" in "The man was bitten by the dog"), and its presence among the words to be unscrambled eliminates this challenge. Similarly, part of what is challenging about negated sentences is the frequent need to insert the auxiliary verb "do" in the appropriate tense, which is already done for you in examples like "the keys", "the girl", "her pocket", "put", "did not", "in". The presence of an appropriately tensed auxiliary verb and an appropriately un-tensed main verb similarly give away much of what is challenging about the syntax of questions.

Many of the more challenging syntactic structures, particularly structures involving various sorts of embedded clauses, turn out to be similarly difficult to elicit in ways that do not give away parts of the answer. There is therefore a significant limit on the ability of these tests, either singularly or collectively, to assess the more advanced grammar skills: skills that may be especially lacking in children with language deficits. These children may therefore eventually achieve ceiling scores on the standard grammar tests, but with their remaining deficits going unrecognized and unremediated, even as these deficits subtly affect their performance in school and beyond.

In addition to concerns about how comprehensive these grammar assessments are, there is the issue of time consumption. Language assessments can take several hours to administer and score, and the IPSyn, in particular, may take even longer to transcribe and codify. This gives us all the more reason to consider whether any components of the assessment process could instead be performed by linguistic technology.

Easiest to automate are the receptive grammar assessments, all of which, as we saw, involve giving the child a specific, predetermined verbal prompt and having the child select the corresponding picture from a predetermined set. As we will see in the next section, this sort of protocol has already been automated in the context of receptive language instruction.

Productive language assessments are more challenging to automate. As far as the IPSyn goes, a combination of speech recognition software and automatic parsing might substitute for much of the examiner's role, which, as we saw, involves recording 100 utterances of spontaneous speech and then transcribing and analyzing them for particular grammatical features. Recently, software has been developed that attempts to automate this last step. However, given that spontaneous speech is often syntactically messy, with lots of pauses, repetitions, and false starts (when the speaker interrupts his or her sentence and starts over again), these automatic ratings are complicated to execute and imperfect in their accuracy. The computerized profiling (CP), of Long, Fey and Channell (2004), for example, while it calculates IPSyn scores automatically, turns out in practice to be unreliable, particularly for older children, whose utterances tend to be more syntactically complex. The CP, therefore, is used only as a first pass, and its analysis is corrected manually. Another automated scorer of IPSyn transcripts is the ac105-IPSyn (Lavie, MacWhinney & Sagae 2005). This takes as its input transcripts that have been annotated using a system that, among other things, demarcates the various disfluencies of spontaneous speech: namely, the CHILDES syntactic annotation scheme. It then uses existing linguistic processing tools to remove disfluencies, analyze the utterances morphologically, and tag parts of speech. The result is run through a parser and the output is then used to obtain IPSyn scores. In their own efficacy testing, Lavie, MacWhinney and Sagae (2005) find their scores to be quite close to scores that were computed manually. Independent efficacy testing, perhaps accompanied by further refinements, is necessary before the ac105-IPSyn is ready to take over from humans.

Also, for all that the ac105-IPSyn has automated, transcripts still need to be generated and annotated by hand. In principle, a tool could be developed that does this transcription automatically. Add in a speech recognizer, and the entire process could then be automated. Although this may be a long way off, it would substantially improve the power of the IPSyn. Currently, it takes many man-hours to manually transcribe and annotate a sample of 100 utterances. Full automation would make it practicable to sample much larger quantities of child speech, allowing for a much more accurate measure of the range of syntactic structures in the child's productive repertoire – including a number of complex structures that IPSyn's index currently omits. Given that the more complex structures tend to occur less frequently, not only would such a widened sampling increase the accuracy of the IPSyn; it would also extend its usability to students who are more linguistically advanced than the pre-K children it currently assesses. If sufficiently accurate and comprehensive in its discrimination of syntactic complexity, an automated IPSyn could also analyze writing samples, providing a separate score for productive syntax in writing, thereby showing relative strengths and weaknesses, anticipating difficulties with classroom writing assignments, and providing yet more robust linguistic profiling.

What about the elicitation of specific syntactic structures that we saw in the productive grammar subtests of the CELF and CASL? Might a computerized version of these tests overcome some of their shortcomings? A rigid computer algorithm that prompts students with pictures and automatically and consistently constrains their responses might indeed outperform human testers in compelling subjects to use particular structures. In eliciting a passive sentence to describe a dog biting a man, for example, an automated program could repeatedly output "Please start with the word 'man'" until the child complies, and it could supply only certain, specific word buttons to click on, making it impossible to input non-passive descriptions like "The man was hurt after the dog bit him". On the other hand, the program could overcome the Sentence Assembly's shortcoming of giving away crucial word forms by including all word forms that the child might conceivably choose – for example, in addition to "bitten" in the above example, "bite", "bites", "biting", and "bit". In principle, such comprehensive word lists could also be used in a therapist-administered assessment. But given the dozens of words that these lists must sometimes contain and that the child, in turn, must keep track of and manipulate, a software-based interface potentially offers a more user friendly medium.

Comprehensive word lists in a software-based medium are one of the key features of GrammarTrainer, a computerized, productive grammar teaching program to be discussed in the next section. As we will see, GrammarTrainer already has the mechanisms in place to elicit the gamut of fundamental grammatical structures of English and to automatically assess those structures for correctness. Also, its step-by-step feedback allows it to analyze, one by one, different types of errors. In fact, a GrammarTrainer-based pilot test has been developed for the purpose of placing learners within the curriculum. It uses a complex algorithm that automatically advances or retreats from level to level depending on the correctness of the user's answers, gradually zeroing in on a particular placement level. This test could, in principle, be tweaked and normed for general placement purposes, particularly with the addition of text-to-speech (TTS) and speech-recognition components that obviate the need for users to recognize written words on buttons. The one big limitation to this assessment methodology as it currently exists is that it does not assess spoken input – only text-based input via word buttons.

Let us turn, finally, to the assessment of the phonemic awareness deficits that underlie dyslexia. Traditional tests of phonological processing (e.g. Stanovich, Cunningham & Cramer 1984) have the examiner orally presenting various words or syllables and then asking the child to recognize or manipulate their phonemes in various ways – say by identifying words or syllables that share initial or final consonants or medial vowels, or by altering those initial or final consonants or medial vowels to create new words or syllables. Cassady, Smith and Lind (2005) have noted that this oral test delivery may be compromised by the particular accents of examiners. They discuss a program that uses standardized, pre-recorded speech. A more refined computerized assessment might slow down the recorded sounds and exaggerate the transitions between them. This is the strategy used in Fast ForWord, a linguistic software program, discussed in the next section, that provides phonological awareness training. Slowing down speech sounds and exaggerating speech sound transitions would help gauge the degree to which children with phonemic processing difficulties need these adjustments as a starting point for remediation. Add in a speech recognizer, and the entire assessment process could be automated – except that the recognizer would have to be sophisticated enough to process child speech (notoriously difficult for today's recognizers) and to recognize subtle phonological errors.

3.2 Linguistic technologies for remediation

Linguistic software shows promise, not only in assessing students' language skills, but also in providing remediation. A generation ago, prior to advancements in linguistic technology, language remediation was limited to in-person sessions with speech/language therapists. Traditional speech/language therapy, of course, remains an invaluable component of language remediation (and of speech remediation in particular, which, recall is outside the scope of this book). However, it also entails certain challenges that software programs can ameliorate. In-person therapy is labor intensive, expensive, and often inadequately covered by insurance, and, when it occurs in a clinical rather than a school setting, can involve substantial commute times for parents and children. Its frequency, limited by all these factors, is typically a mere one to two hours per week.

Moreover, while in-person speech/language therapy can be a highly effective venue for teaching everyday vocabulary and idioms, and especially the real-life social aspects of language (pragmatics, conversational dynamics), there is one key aspect of language to which, as things currently stand, it is less suited: namely, grammar. In large part, this is the result of what traditional speech/language training programs can realistically cover. A full survey of a language's grammatical structures would probably require several courses specifically devoted to grammar, with many weeks examining the more complex rules – for example, the rules for forming questions or for choosing among different verb forms ("chased", "was chasing", "has chased", "had chased", "will chase", "would chase", "will chase", "will have chased", "would have chased", etc.) or for forming relative clauses ("The boy who was chasing the dog"; "The dog that the boy was chasing") and other embedded clauses ("The boy is hard for the dog to chase"). The field of syntax pedagogy, furthermore, is still underdeveloped, leaving speech/language therapists with little guidance on how to teach the more complicated rules.

Even certain aspects of pragmatics elude traditional speech/language therapy: namely, the distinctions among first, second, and third person pronouns ("I" vs. "you" vs. "he"/"she'). Difficulty in making this distinction, seen frequently in autism, has been attributed to a more general difficulty with perspective taking. Figuring out on your own, as typically developing children do, that "I" and "me" refer to whoever is speaking, that "you" refers to whoever is being addressed, and that third person pronouns ("she", "him", "they", etc.) refer to people who are neither speaking nor being addressed, involves putting yourself in the shoes of other speakers and figuring out who they are addressing and who they are referring to. Such perspective taking skills require cognitive flexibility and are difficult to teach. The alternative, teaching "I", "you", "he", etc., directly as regular vocabulary words, is also quite difficult. Showing the child illustrative pictures – pictures of one character addressing another character while a third character looks on – presupposes that the child can put himself in the characters' shoes; in other words, that he already has perspective taking skills. Correcting the child's mistakes in real-life interactions involves a similar chicken-and-egg problem. Suppose the child says, "You want juice" when he or she actually means "I want juice". If you correct the child by saying "*You* want juice", you might sound like you are simply agreeing with what he or she said. If you say, "*No, you* want juice" you might sound incoherent. If you instead correct the child by saying "*I* want juice" or "No, *I* want juice", then you are, literally, making the same pronoun error that the child is making. Either type of correction risks reinforcing the child's error – especially because interpreting the error message correctly involves the same kind of perspective taking skills that are lacking in the first place.

Unfortunately, there are no established, linguistically informed, teaching-oriented textbooks that would assist therapists in addressing these topics in grammar and pronoun pragmatics. Indeed, vis-à-vis the fundamentals of grammar, existing speech/language curricula are woefully incomplete and imprecise.

Let us consider, for example, one major therapeutic approach to autism in particular, Applied Behavioral Analysis. This approach, using a behaviorist training protocol to which children with autism are often especially responsive, has been quite successful in teaching a number of non-linguistic tasks. But with linguistic instruction, ABA falls short. Limiting its approach to language is a reductionist scheme developed by B. F. Skinner that has been completely supplanted by modern linguistics (see Hurewitz & Beals 2008). As such, it fails to address the rules that govern how words fit together into longer utterances, and restricts learning to the memorization of scripted responses and patterns that do not generalize to arbitrary linguistic utterances. Consider, for example, the lesson on wh-questions in Teach Me Language (Freeman & Dake 1997), an ABA-based language curriculum. Here we find "A thing answers a WHAT question" and "A person answers a WHO question", but nothing more precise about what a "thing" is, let alone what a "question" is, let alone what it means to "answer" a question. Nor do we find any information about the syntax of wh-questions, which, as in "Who did you see?", involves an auxiliary verb ("do"), the shifting of tense from the main verb to the auxiliary verb ("you saw" → "you did see"), and subject-auxiliary inversion ("you did see" → "did you see").

Diametrically opposed to ABA's behaviorist approach to language therapy, but at least as inadequate and as uninformed by modern linguistics, is the Affect Based Language Curriculum (Greenspan & Lewis 2005). This curriculum, based on a conception of autism as a disorder primarily of emotional attachment, and on a conception of language as primarily social rather than grammatical in nature, has even less to say about the details of teaching grammar rules.

Plenty of other grammar teaching materials are available to speech/language therapists, for example, over the web, but they tend to cover only certain of the more basic aspects of grammar rather than offering a comprehensive curriculum. A theme-based package called "Grateful Grammar" for Thanksgiving (Palyu, n.d.), for example, covers "is" vs. "are", "has" vs. "have", sentences with progressive verbs, and irregular past tense, but does not address more complex verb tenses.

The upshot is that few speech/language therapists have the materials they need to teach language-impaired children how to produce the many types of well-formed sentences that deviate – as questions do – from the most basic subject-verb-object structures (sentences like "I want juice" or "The marble is in the basket"). This potentially leaves language impaired children unable to express (or even comprehend) not just questions, but a whole host of complex thoughts: for example, causal statements ("Because X is true, Y is true"), conditional and hypothetical statements ("If X happened, then Y would happen"; "If X were to happen, then Y would happen"), statements expressing how one thing depends on another ("The more you practice, the better you will do"), and statements about other statements ("Sally thinks that the marble is in the basket, but she is wrong").

Computerized instruction potentially bypasses many of these in-person teaching limitations. While computerized language curricula are not cheap, some programs costing many hundreds of dollars, when divided by the number of hours of use a child can get from them, they are far less expensive, per hour, than in-person speech therapy is. Conveniently portable into homes, schools, and speech therapy clinics, they involve far less overhead per session. Furthermore, provided they are sufficiently linguistically informed, they can potentially deploy and disseminate broadly the linguistic expertise in complex areas like grammar, which, as we have discussed, is unrealistic to expect of traditional in-person therapy.

For all these benefits, there remain certain key aspects of language that are not suitable to computerized instruction and are in fact much *more* suited to traditional, in-person therapy. Vocabulary is one example. Computers are limited in their ability to convey word meaning. They can show pictures and animations of words with easily depicted meanings. But the overwhelming majority of words are not easily and unambiguously depicted. Consider how many of the words inside this paragraph, for example, cannot be illustrated in pictures. Even depictions that might seem clear to neurotypical children risk leading children with autism astray. Children with autism are inherently under-aware of communicative intent, and thus of the communicative intent behind pictures in particular. Some children will focus on small details or elements relating to special interests rather than the big picture or its most salient element(s). As a result, they may make what are called "associative mapping errors" (see Bloom 2002). These are errors that involve mapping a word to whatever one happens to be focusing on at the time the word was presented. So, for example, a picture of a boy painting, used to illustrate the meaning of the verb "paint", might induce a child who is obsessed with colors to map the word "paint" instead to the particular shade of green of the paint that the boy happens to be using.

Instead of conveying word meanings through pictures, why not convey them through words? But definitions and usages show only how words relate to one another (as, for example, the word "president" relates to the words "leader" and "country"), not how they relate to the real world. If you do not already know what a "leader" and a "country" are, you still will not know what a "president" is. Even basic words are problematic: the definitions of simple words like "boy" often contain terminology that is more advanced ("young", "male") and words with irreducible meanings like "joy" elude definition altogether.

There are, in short, serious limitations on the ability of computers to teach vocabulary, particularly to children on the autism spectrum who, because of their tendencies toward mapping errors, require careful monitoring. Only a real-life teacher or therapist can guide the child interactively through the often subtle ways in which a particular word relates to the world, watching for signs of confusion or comprehension and clarifying things accordingly. Only a real-life teacher or therapist can discriminate among the different aspects of an object to which a given word might refer. Consider, for example, a word used in reference to a fuzzy, round, yellowish orange object in a bowl: that word might refer to its type (e.g. if the word used is "peach"), its more general category (if the word used is "fruit"), its exterior ("skin"), the texture of this exterior ("fuzzy"), its deeper texture ("soft"), its color ("yellowish orange"), its shape ("round"), or its condition ("ripe"). As for the abstract words that comprise the majority of all words – for example, "abstract", "comprise", and "majority" – only real-life teachers and real-life experiences can guide a child, interactively, toward understanding and eventual mastery.

Another key aspect of language to which computers are ill suited – and which is also a key deficit area in autism – is pragmatics. The component of language that depends on the presumed intentions of particular speakers along with the presumed knowledge of particular listeners, pragmatics encompasses an open-ended array of ever-changing real-world situations, representative samples of which are extremely difficult to simulate on screen or to anticipate and generate automatically. Pragmatics is what accounts, for example, for the variability of what the utterance "It's brilliant" can convey: is the speaker using it to describe a bright light, an idea she finds ingenious, or an idea that is clearly ridiculous? Pragmatics is what determines whether a speaker should refer to a light as "a light" or "the light", and pragmatics is what determines what additional, unstated messages are conveyed by particular utterances in particular contexts. For example, "It's dark inside" conveys anything from "Please turn on the light" to "It looks like no one is home". The range of possible situations and possible usages is too large and too elusive for a pedagogically principled sequence of computerized simulations that are not excessive in number and yet still manage to teach skills that generalize to real-world interactions. And the open-ended nature of possible correct responses to any given situation or simulation makes it difficult for a program even to assess which user responses are pragmatically felicitous – let alone to give appropriate feedback.

One recent anecdotal account (see Newman 2014) of a boy with autism suggests one way in which a computerized medium can provide a venue at least for pragmatics practice (as opposed to pragmatics instruction) – specifically, practice with conversational pragmatics, or appropriate conversational utterances. The program in question is Siri, an iPhone app that, manifesting itself as a disembodied female voice, functions as a personal assistant and Internet navigator, adapting to the user's idiosyncratic language usage and queries. In this boy's experience, Siri provides a tolerant, safe environment for carrying on a conversation – and thus for practicing his conversational skills. However, for all Siri's linguistic programming, she does not provide explicit feedback about pragmatic appropriateness – only the implicit feedback that comes from the degree to which her responses match the user's expectations. Given that Siri's own linguistic comprehension and conversational skills are notoriously far from perfect, there is a limit to how reliable and useful her feedback can be. Nonetheless, as programs like Siri become more sophisticated, they potentially offer an increasingly effective medium for the practice and implicit learning of conversational skills.

Another type of program that might provide such practice, but in a more constrained way, are dialog systems. Described in detail in Chapter 1, these are systems that use speech recognition and natural language understanding technologies to give conversationally appropriate responses to a user's spoken utterances. These systems use dialog management tools to control the conversational back and forth, and in the case of structured dialog applications, the conversational goals as well. Dialog systems can thus provide feedback about pragmatic appropriateness, responding in ways that the user did or did not anticipate – and in ways that, while more constrained than in real-life interactions, are perhaps more reliable than Siri. In addition to this immediate feedback, the system can provide feedback about the user's progress over time: as discussed in Chapter 1, dialog systems can potentially record the length of users' utterances, the number of conversational slots they fill, and the latency between the end of the system's utterances and the beginning of the users' utterances. Perhaps most importantly, as with Siri, dialog systems allow those with pragmatic impairments a lower-stress way to practice conversation skills than that offered by real-life humans.

There are thus some potential avenues for practice, and for incidental learning, in conversational pragmatics. But when it comes to direct instruction and systematic feedback in this and other open-ended, context-dependent aspects of pragmatics, effective computerized training programs remain elusive.

The exception to all this is a small subset of pragmatics involving certain usages that are systematically constrained and relatively independent of specific situations. Examples include conventionalized indirect requests like "Can you pass the salt?", which, even though literally it queries the addressee's ability to pass the salt, almost always is uttered as a request for salt. Other examples of conventionalized non-literal usages are idioms like "Give me a hand" and "cry one's eyes out" and conventional metaphors like "Time is money" and "Time is running out". Some people (see, for example, Happé 1995) have cited such usages as canonical examples of the difficulty that figurative language poses to children with autism. But what is most problematic for such children are not these cases, with their fixed, easily memorized meanings. What is most problematic, rather, are instances of figurative language and indirect language that are not so common and conventional (like "chase down that idea" or "salt?", which can be either a request or an offer), as well as utterances that are possibly ironic (as discussed above with "It's brilliant"). Conventionalized figurative uses ("Can you pass the salt?", "cry one's eyes out", etc.) can be taught in the same direct way that vocabulary words are – but, as with many vocabulary words, they may well turn out to be too difficult to depict and instruct via computer.

Other context-free elements of pragmatics are so-called generalized implicatures. These include "some people" implying "not all people" and "He thinks it's cold out", implying "He does not know it is cold out". This kind of implicature may be possible to depict schematically, i.e. abstracted from particular contexts. It may therefore lend itself to systematic, context-independent exercises, for which, as we will discuss below, computer software programs are particularly well suited.

Similarly systematic are so-called deictics: words whose meanings are a function of formal differences in speaker vs. listener perspectives. The first vs. second vs. third person pronouns we discussed earlier, challenging though they are to children on the autism spectrum, have this characteristic: "I" always referring to the speaker; "you", to the addressee, and third person pronouns (e.g. "he", "she", and "they"), to third parties. Other examples of deictics are "here" and "this" (near the speaker) vs. "there" and "that" (further away from the speaker) and "come" (movement toward the speaker) vs. "go" (movement away from the speaker). These sorts of regular patterns also lend themselves to systematic, schematic computer-based exercises, even in the case of the pronoun distinctions that, as we saw above, elude traditional in-person therapy. Indeed, as we will discuss below, a systematic, repetitive software-based approach may be the most effective way to teach these key pronoun distinctions to the learners with autism who struggle with them.

This brings us to the one key component of language that is ideally suited to computerized instruction, namely, grammar. The rules of grammar, which generate the countless possible sentences that make up a language, are, for all intents and purposes, fully independent of the real world. While the words and their meanings will change based on context, the rules for putting them in the correct order with the correct endings attached remain constant. While what a sentence conveys will change depending on context, the rules for constructing that sentence remain constant. And those rules – which in English include the above-discussed algorithm for question formation (do-insertion, tense shifting, and subject-auxiliary inversion) – are not only decontextualized, but also finite in number and, however complex they may be, highly regular. In short, unlike most vocabulary words and most of pragmatics, grammar rules are ideally suited to the logical automaticity of computer programs.

While grammar might appear to be just one of just three key components of language – a sister to word meaning and pragmatics – it is arguably the most central. Grammar is the bridge between individual words and pragmatic utterances. Grammar is what distinguishes the limited Pidgin language of 2-year-olds and other beginners from the fully expressive language of older fluent speakers. And grammar is what allows speakers (and writers) to move beyond simple and highly context-dependent communication about the here and now ("Mommy cookie") to communication that is liberated from the immediate context: communication about situations that may be long over or merely possible, hypothetical, or desirable ("Mommy had a cookie"; "Does Mommy have a cookie?"; "I want you to give me a cookie"; "Earlier, I thought that Mommy had a cookie"). Grammar also facilitates thinking: research has shown grammar mastery to underlie the ability not just to communicate about hypothetical situations and alternative perspectives on reality and to understand such communications, but also to entertain thoughts about hypothetical situations and alternative perspectives (see, for example, de Villiers & de Villiers 2003). In short, grammar is what allows both the conception of, and communication about, arbitrary, arbitrarily complex thoughts; thoughts about the world as it is, might be, ought to be, and as different people conceive it to be. The fact that grammar is so conducive to computerized instruction, and that computerized instruction may be a better way for those with language impairments to learn grammar rules than in-person instruction can realistically be, means that computers potentially play a tremendous role in assisting in the remediation of language deficits – especially since many of these deficits, as we have seen, specifically involve deficits in grammar.

Another aspect of language that linguistic software is poised to teach is phonemic awareness, or the ability to process language at the level of the consonants and vowels that form its phonological building blocks. A deficit in phonemic awareness, as discussed in Chapter 2, is one of the two core deficits of dyslexia. Some researchers have proposed that phonemic awareness can be boosted by slowing down the sounds of words and syllables and exaggerating the transitions from one phoneme to the next (see, for example, Rogowsky, Papamichalis, Villa, Heim & Tallal 2013). Precisely this technique is used by one of the language teaching software programs discussed below.

Throughout this survey of what linguistic technology potentially can and cannot offer to language-impaired children, we have seen time and again that that which most eludes in-person therapy is conducive to linguistic technology and that which most eludes linguistic technology is conducive to in-person therapy. In particular, the real-world aspects of word meaning and pragmatics that surpass the computational capabilities of computer technologies are handled effectively, and routinely, by traditional speech/language therapists. And the formal rules of grammar and conventionalized pragmatics that, in all their abstract complexity, surpass the linguistic and pedagogical resources of traditional speech/language therapies can, at least in principle, be handled by computer technologies. The same is true of the acoustic manipulation of speech sounds discussed above for phonemic awareness training. In short, when it comes to language remediation, it turns out that computer technologies and human therapists are perfect complements.

In complementing speech/language therapy, computer-based instruction offers some additional, pedagogical benefits. In particular, it can optimize three key components of the learning environment: zone of proximal development (ZPD) instruction, drill/practice, and immediate feedback. ZPD refers to the zone just between a student's current level of mastery and what he or she can do only with help from others. Some research suggests that students progress most quickly if consistently given work just above their current level of mastery (see, for example, Kulik, Kulik & Bangert-Drowns 1990; Engelmann 1999). Drill/ practice, for its part, is instrumental to attaining mastery, with different students needing different amounts depending on how frequently they err. As for feedback, its benefits have emerged from several studies of computer-based learning. Mason and Bruning (2001) find that both the immediate and the delayed achievement outcomes among students using computer-based instruction are generally greater for those who also receive feedback. Smith et al. (2013) find that implicit category learning depends on immediate feedback. Quick, regular, consistent feedback also deters students from mislearning from repeated errors. Finally, where negative feedback is concerned, feedback that analyzes responses and highlights which components of a response are wrong turns learner errors into teachable moments. Indeed, several studies (Roper 1977; Waldrop, Justen & Adams 1986; Pridemore & Klein 1991; Whyte, Karolick, Neilsen, Elder & Hawley 1995) find that feedback containing more elaborative information produced increased understanding. In particular, both Waldrop et al. (1986) and Pridemore and Klein (1991) found response-contingent feedback to be significantly more effective than simple, right-or-wrong feedback. What all these studies collectively suggest, then, is that learning is optimized in environments that provide immediate, elaborated feedback.

When it comes to grammar learning in particular, where mastery is thought to be optimized by implicit learning in the basal ganglia (Ullman et al. 1997), there is some evidence that right-or-wrong feedback is sufficient for learning. However, right-or-wrong feedback and elaborative feedback are mutually compatible: elaborative feedback can break a user's response into components and give right-or-wrong feedback on each component. As we will see below, this is how feedback works in the GrammarTrainer program.

Indeed, software programs, particularly those that perform linguistic analyses on user responses, can readily optimize all three of these pedagogical goals. In terms of ZPD learning, computerized instruction allows customizable level setting and lesson delivery at each student's unique level and learning pace. Given the tremendous heterogeneity in the severity of deficits and responses to treatment both across and within the various language disorders, such customizability benefits everyone. Further optimizing ZPD learning, computer programs potentially allow a seamless integration of assessment and remediation, with built-in pretests leading automatically to initial placements, with ongoing progress tests interacting, or even overlapping, with lesson delivery, with lesson advancement dynamically tailored to progress, with automatic remediation delivered as needed, and with initial, ongoing, and final assessments made available to real-life supervisors. Down at the level of individual exercises, answer-revealing prompts can be highlighted at first, promoting error-free learning, and then gradually faded as the user progresses toward mastery.

In terms of drill/practice, computer software offers unlimited opportunities. Programs can patiently recycle through exercises whenever a student's progress stalls. They can reshuffle these exercises randomly, such that students with strengths in rote memorization (common in autism) do not end up simply memorizing sequences of answers. And they can automatically identify which exercises are more frequently mis-answered and shuffle these in more frequently.

In terms of feedback, computerized instruction can readily automate the kinds of consistent and immediate feedback that steers students toward correct answers and prevents errors from becoming habitual. Additionally, a well-designed linguistic processing program can provide elaborative feedback, giving users accurate, linguistically informed information about why their answers are wrong, and thus turning errors into teachable moments – and eliciting self-corrections that may further enhance learning.

Computer software also readily automates the process of record keeping, with the capacity to collect and store information about each user's sessions and create detailed data reports on progress, complete with statistical analysis and user-friendly graphical representations.

In practice, computerized learning in autism has shown promise, leading in some cases to increased learning as compared to more standard human-to-human instruction (Xin & Jitendra 1999; Moore & Calvert 2000; Bosseler & Massaro 2003). The case is less clear with other language impairments (see Bishop, Adams & Rosen 2006), although there is some evidence (see below) that computerized training of phonemic awareness can help students with dyslexia or auditory processing disorders.

When it comes to autism in particular, research has found that some learners find interactions with computers less stressful and more engaging than interactions with people (Chen & Bernard-Opitz 1993; Heimann, Nelson, Tjus & Gillberg 1995). Furthermore, compared with the natural environment, computer-assisted instruction bypasses some of the obstacles that may prevent children on the autism spectrum from acquiring full language in the first place – for example, diminished tendencies to orient to speech sounds and to observe other people and what they are communicating (see Chapter 2 for more discussion). These weaknesses may limit the efficacy of traditional face-to-face communication therapies in treating clients with autism. Computerized delivery of language, on the other hand, exposes users to language without requiring social attention or interaction. Thus, for those aspects of language that best lend themselves to computerized instruction, linguistic software programs may offer clients with autism a learning environment that bypasses the challenges of live speech and social attention that may be responsible in part for their language delays.

Furthermore, while live speech is fleeting, often rapid, and hard to "replay", the cues and prompts within linguistic software environments are easily repeated or slowed down – a benefit for the many learners whose language challenges stem, in part, from difficulties in sustaining attention or in processing speech sounds.

3.2.1 Programs that address phonological processing

Turning to what there exists in the way of established, computerized remediation programs, we begin with dyslexia. Dyslexia, as we have discussed, is largely a disorder of phonological processing. Specifically aimed at this disorder are certain units of a well-known linguistic software curriculum known as Fast ForWord. These units present phonological processing exercises in which users wear headphones and attend to recordings of speech sounds that (as mentioned in our earlier discussion) have been slowed down and modified so as to amplify their most rapidly changing acoustic features. The idea is to highlight the distinctions among such similar sounds as "ba", "da", or "ta" and then gradually to fade the exaggerations such that the student becomes more aware of the distinguishing phonemes (here "b", "d", and "t"), even in everyday, unmodified speech, and eventually acquires the phonemic awareness needed to decode written words fluently.

Such a training protocol sounds promising, but how efficacious has it proved to be? Non-randomized studies (Heim et al. 2013; Rogowsky et al. 2013) conducted by researchers affiliated with Fast ForWord have found that the training produces gains in language and literacy. But randomized controlled studies have generally shown it to be ineffective, especially in terms of reading skills. A systematic meta-analysis of all randomized controlled trials concluded that there is no evidence for efficacy in reducing impairments in reading and oral learning (Strong, Torgerson, Torgerson & Hulme 2011). Possibly, the software does improve phonological awareness somewhat – but not enough to produce measurable, lasting improvements in reading. Indeed, Heim et al. (2013) observe pre- and post-training EEG measurements that they suggest may show that "specific aspects of inefficient sensory processing are ameliorated after training". One could further explore the effects of training on processing via the phonological processing assessments described in Section 3.1, in which students have to recognize and manipulate phonemes. If such assessments show post-training improvements, one could next explore what additional training protocols might boost or supplement these gains enough to produce measurable improvements in reading.

Speech recognition technology suggests one possibility. A speech recognizer could potentially supplement Fast ForWord's passive discrimination exercises with exercises in which users actively manipulate phonemes – practicing the kinds of phonemic manipulations used to gauge phonemic awareness in the first place. Users could be asked to produce syllables that rhyme with a given syllable or that start or end with different consonant sounds, and the speech recognizer could enable appropriate feedback. However, given that children's speech is particularly challenging for speech recognizers (see Chapter 1), especially the often poorly articulated speech of children with language impairments, and that the recognizer would have to make the same, fine phonological distinctions that the child is being asked to make, only the most sensitive of speech recognizers might be up to this task.

The ultimate goal of any phonological training program, of course, and the ultimate outcome that efficacy studies of such programs should look for, are decoding skills that are fluent enough to eliminate bottlenecks to higher-level reading comprehension.

3.2.2 Programs that address comprehension, or receptive language

We turn now to programs that address comprehension, or receptive language. As discussed in Chapter 2, receptive language problems are quite widespread, affecting a subgroup of children with SLI, as well as children with autism and children with general language impairments.

Comprehension, at its most basic, operates at the level of individual words. Here, comprehension skills, essentially, are vocabulary skills. And even though vocabulary is often a relative strength in both autism and SLI, many children with moderate to severe autism still experience serious impairments, even in understanding basic words. The same is true of children with general language delays. We begin, therefore, by looking at programs that teach word meanings – keeping in mind the various challenges for computerized vocabulary instruction we have already discussed.

There are, as it turns out, a number of established software programs that address vocabulary deficits. These include Cosmo, Fast ForWord (Language and

Language to Reading), Laureate Learning, TeachTown, Timo Stories, Timo Vocabulary, and Milo Speaks. Cosmo, catering to the needs of younger children, covers such basics as concrete adjectives, spatial prepositions, and numbers. Timo Stories focuses on day-to-day vocabulary, taught both in the context of stories and phrases and in terms of their semantic classifications. Milo Speaks, an iPad App, shows illustrative animations of over 100 basic action verbs.

TeachTown and Laureate are particularly comprehensive in their coverage of preschool vocabulary – each of them instructing hundreds of basic terms. Teach-Town organizes content by topic, such as animals, colors, and time. Laureate's various basic-level packages cover hundreds of basic nouns, as well as concrete verbs, adjectives, and spatial prepositions. Figures 3.1 to 3.3 show screenshots from Laureate Learning.

Timo Vocabulary and Fast ForWord's Robo-Dog teach a more specialized and sophisticated vocabulary that is more appropriate for school-aged learners. Timo Vocabulary organizes basic concepts into 22 categories ranging from animal groups ("pride", "school", "gaggle") to weather, with many categories further divided into subcategories. Within the category "animals and habitats", for example, one finds "arctic animals"; within "force and movement", one finds "parts of a bicycle". Fast ForWord's Robo-Dog is similarly specialized, teaching terms from arithmetic, geometry, life science, and earth science.

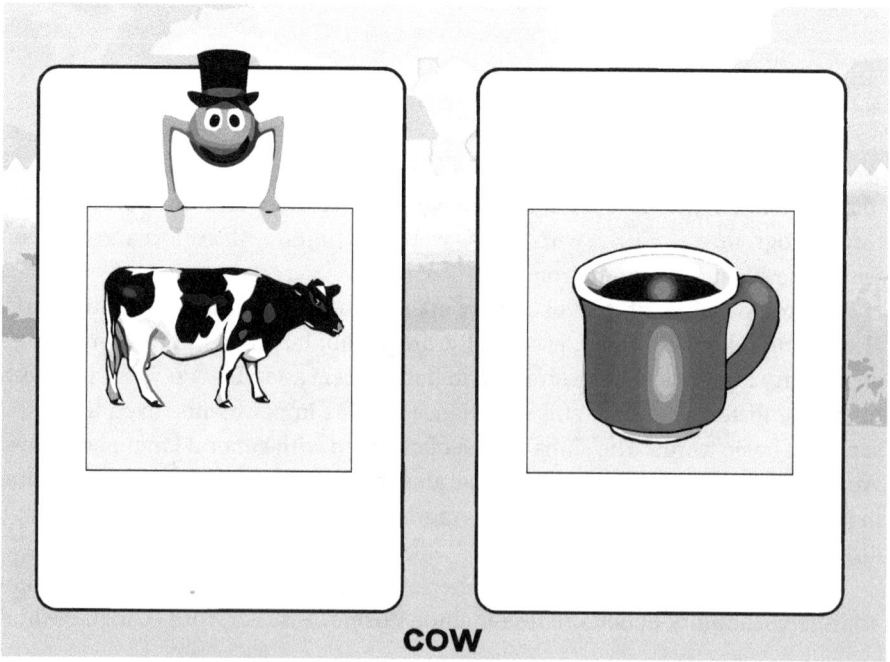

COW

Fig. 3.1: Laureate Learning "First Words".

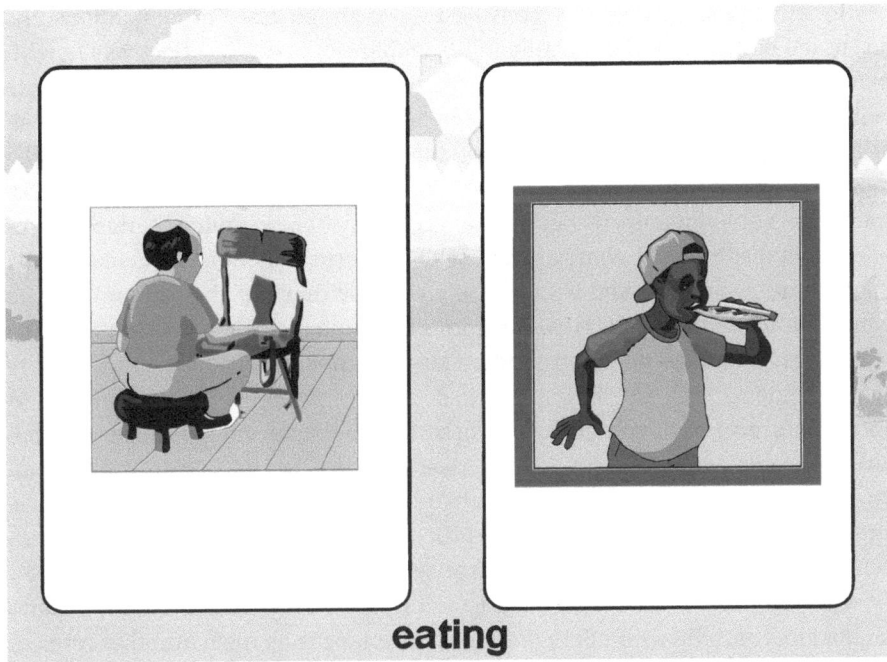

Fig. 3.2: Laureate Learning "First Verbs".

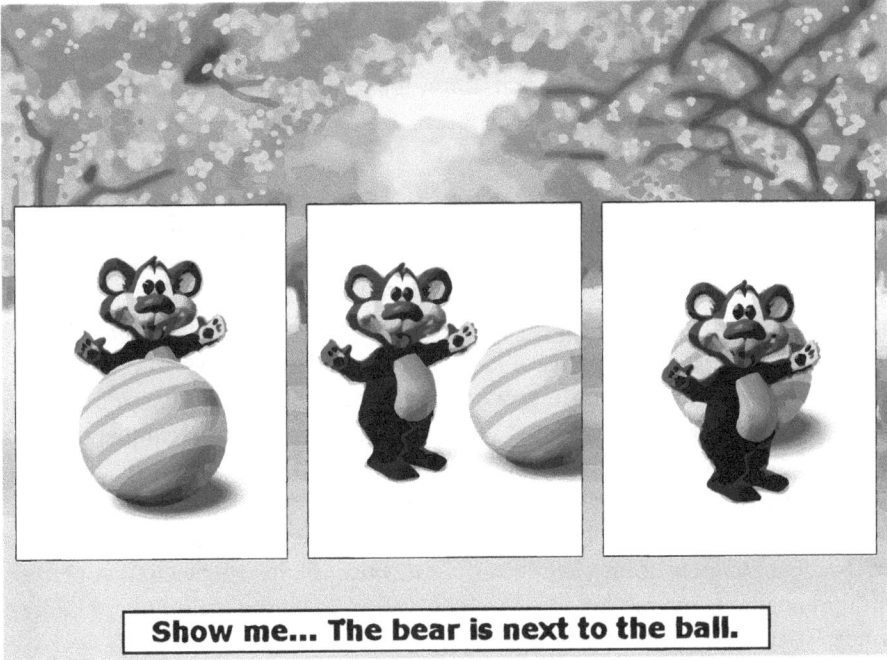

Fig. 3.3: Laureate Learning "Prepositions".

In all cases, meaning is conveyed through pictures or animations. As discussed earlier, this significantly limits which words can be effectively taught: namely, those whose meanings are easily depicted, of which nouns that denote concrete objects or basic geometrical phenomena are the best examples. Consider "table", "ice cream cone", and "rectangle". More abstract words are much more difficult: consider "idea", "think", or "interesting". Most elusive are abstract words that not only cannot be depicted, but whose meanings cannot be isolated from the linguistic contexts in which they occur: function words like "and", "but", "the", and "if". And yet, precisely because they are abstract and hard to depict, words in these latter two categories are often the words with which many moderately language-impaired children struggle the most.

In students with autism in particular, relative strengths and weaknesses in vocabulary do not align with what these picture-based computerized vocabulary programs emphasize. In autism, clear-cut classification, as in the vocabulary categories seen especially in TeachTown and Timo Vocabulary, is a relative strength. What is disproportionately difficult are those terms having to do with mental states ("think", "suspect", "surprised") or social dynamics ("friendship", "love", "authority"). Like other abstract terms, these are quite hard to depict, and for the most part the vocabulary programs do not focus on them. Another concern is that, as discussed earlier, children with autism may attend to the wrong features of pictures and, making incorrect mappings between words and pictures, derive inaccurate meanings from training.

One of the biggest advantages of automated instruction is its ability to store user data and produce detailed reports of student progress for teachers, therapists, and parents. TeachTown and Timo, for example, provide comprehensive data about the level of mastery of specific modules. Cosmo provides linguistically informed descriptions for each module, further clarifying what the child has, and has yet, to master.

Moving beyond the apparent strengths and shortcomings of these various programs, what evidence do we have of actual efficacy? A study of Baldi, an early version of Timo Vocabulary (Bosseler & Massaro 2003) found that eight 7- to 12-year-olds with autism made post-training progress on tests of vocabulary. And a study of TeachTown (Whalen et al. 2010) found that children in preschool to first grade with autism made improvements on general language measures. Both studies included authors affiliated with the respective software companies. The Baldi study, furthermore, lacked control subjects, and the TeachTown study was confounded by the fact that the training included additional offline activities. Nonetheless, these and other vocabulary training programs may well be effective in teaching concrete nouns, action verbs, adjectives expressing visual properties, and prepositions expressing visual relationships, to young children, or children whose vocabulary deficits are fairly severe.

Moving beyond individual words, we reach sentence-level phenomena, particularly grammar and pragmatics. Here, deficits in comprehension, or receptive language, are common not just in children with autism and children with general language delays, but also in a subset of children with SLI.

Beginning here and continuing into the next section, it is grammar in particular that we will focus on, central as it is to language, to the needs of students with autism and SLI, and, finally, to the curriculum of most of those language programs that extend beyond vocabulary. In this section, our focus continues, furthermore, to be on receptive language, and on programs that teach comprehension; programs for productive language, or how to construct well-formed sentences, are discussed in the next section.

The most widely used programs for receptive language at the sentence level, and receptive grammar in particular, are Laureate Learning, Fast ForWord, and HearBuilder. In all three programs, the user is presented with canned (pre-recorded or pre-written) verbal prompts along with sets of pictures or animations to click on or otherwise manipulate in response. For example, the user might be prompted with "The mother is washing the baby" and presented with a set of pictures to choose from (see Fig. 3.4). Alternatively, the user might be presented with a single picture of an array of colored shapes and prompted to "Move the blue triangle under the red square".

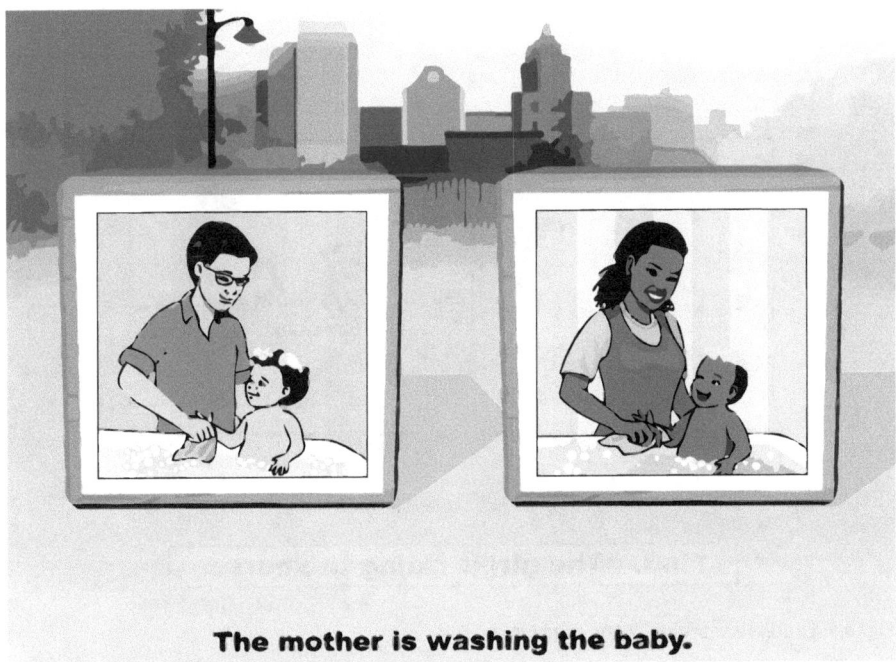

The mother is washing the baby.

Fig. 3.4: Laureate Learning "Simple Sentence Structure".

Thus, in all these programs, the user's tasks only involve comprehending sentences, not constructing them. His responses to prompts, indeed, are consistently non-verbal: he either clicks on one of the picture choices (e.g. the picture in which the mother is washing the baby) or rearranges a single picture by dragging one or more of its elements around the screen (e.g. dragging the blue triangle under the red square).

Most of these programs, dependent as they are on what is easily conveyed through pictures, stick with simple sentence structures. Typical, for example, is Laureate Learning's basic syntax package, Simple Sentence Structure, one example of which we see in Fig. 3.4. Here the user selects from among several pictures the one that matches the subject-verb-object pattern of the sentence. Similar tasks occur in the lower levels of Laureate's Language Links Syntax Assessment and Intervention package. In many of these exercises, for example, Fig. 3.4 or Fig. 3.5 (from Language Links Level 2), one can determine the correct picture by key words alone. In the former, for example, the word "mother" tells you that the second picture is the correct one; in the latter, the giveaway is the word "riding". Attending to the syntax of the sentence, in other words, is not necessary: one does not, for example, need to recognize that "the girl" is the subject of the second sentence and "the horse" is its object.

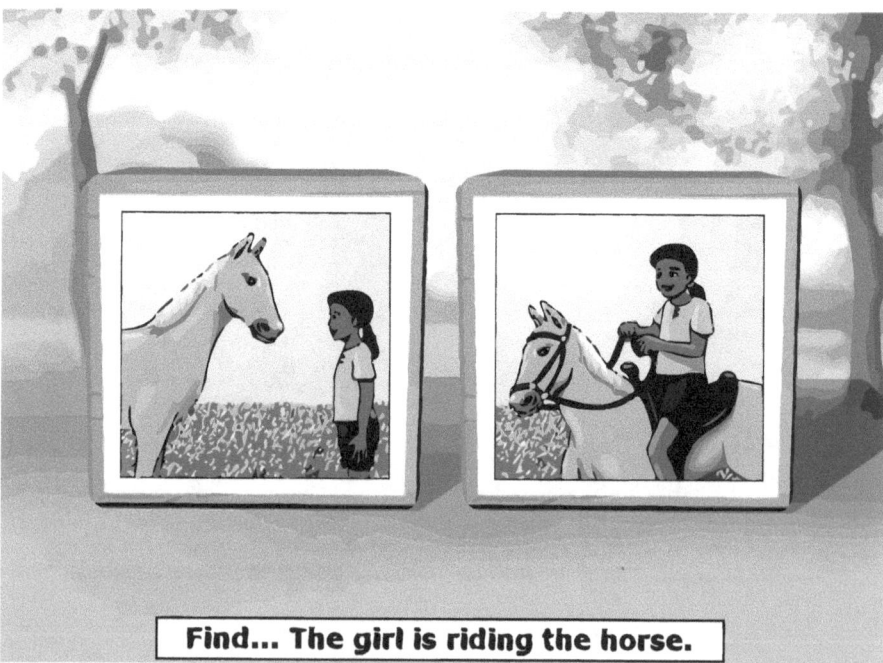

Find... The girl is riding the horse.

Fig. 3.5: Laureate Learning "Language Links 2".

In exercises like these two, rather than requiring the user to make explicit word order distinctions, the program conveys the subject-verb-object pattern by exposing the student to repeated examples of it: repeated examples of subject-verb-object sentences that match pictures in which the subject is the actor and the object is the character being acted upon. While this incidental exposure can lead to learning, the program cannot ensure that it actually does: what, if anything, the user learns depends entirely on whether or not he or she happens to attend to the relevant details. As discussed earlier, users with autism in particular may focus on peripheral details rather than on those that program designers consider most important.

Some of the exercises in these packages do require attention to word order. Consider, for example, Fig. 3.6 from Simple Sentence Structure. Here the picture choices all depict the same nouns ("lion" and "bear") and verb ("riding"), and users must attend to their specific positions in the prompt sentence in order to click on the correct picture. Consistently making the correct selection in exercises like these means learning that the first noun is the subject or actor: the entity that performs the action denoted by the transitive verb.

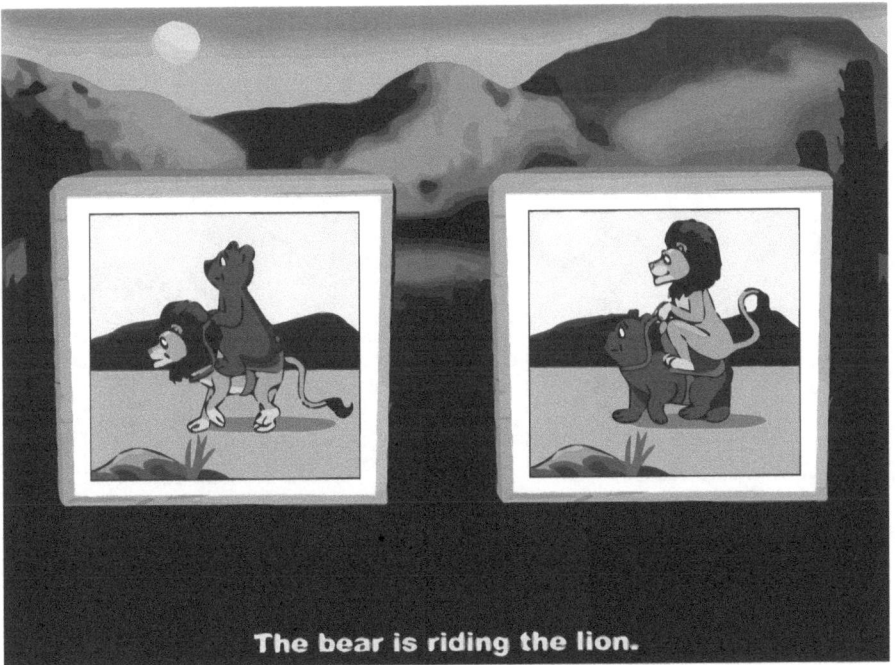

Fig. 3.6: Laureate Learning "Simple Sentence Structure".

Attention to word order is also required by Laureate's passive sentence exercises, found in Language Links Level 6 and seen in Fig. 3.7. As before, both pictures depict the same nouns ("monkey" and "monster") and verb ("washing"), and so word order is once again key. But this time, the first noun in the prompt sentence is the object rather than the subject, and to recognize this, the user must notice such passive markers as the "is" plus past participle "washed" and/or the passive "by"-phrase "by the monkey".

Other structures that deviate from subject-verb-object order are found in the Ele-bot unit of Fast ForWord. Here we find such prompts as "It's the girl that the boy is pushing", where the object ("the girl") precedes the subject ("the boy"). Once again, users must attend, not just to word order, but to specific syntactic markers – "It is ... that ... " – in order to make the correct selection.

Similar attention to detail is required in Laureate's lessons on singular vs. plural verbs, and its lessons on simple past, present progressive, and future verb forms. In the latter set, we find pictures that show – some more clearly than others – actions about to be undertaken, actions in progress, and actions that have already occurred, as in Fig. 3.8. Note that, while it is clear from the set as a

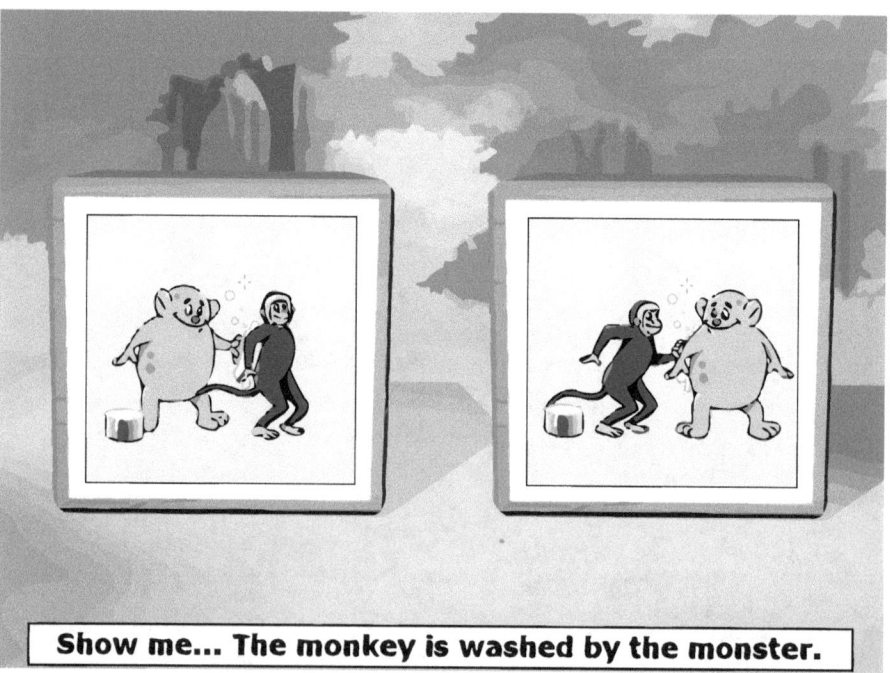

Show me... The monkey is washed by the monster.

Fig. 3.7: Laureate Learning "Language Links 6".

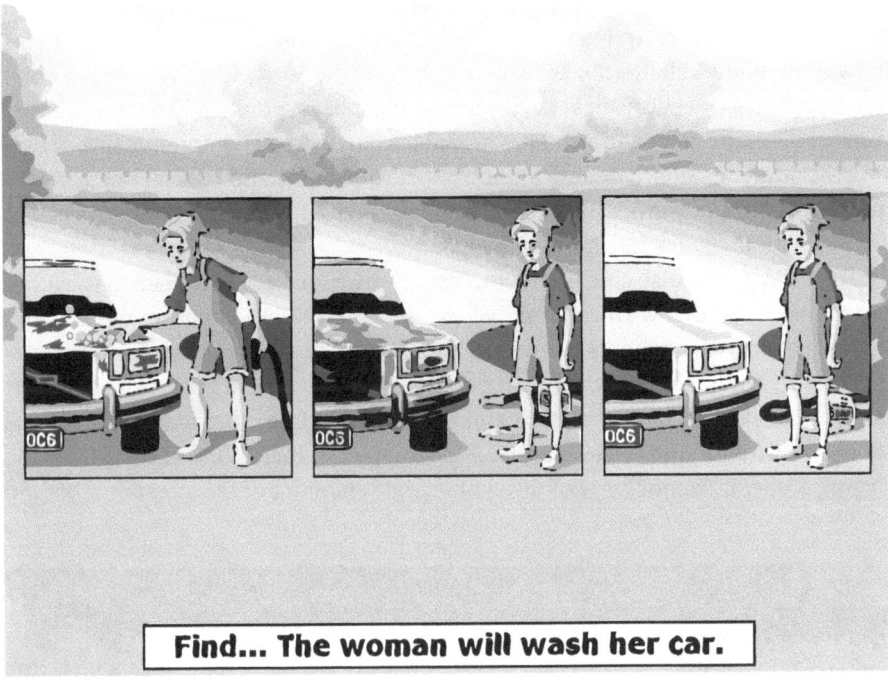

Fig. 3.8: Laureate Learning "Language Links 5".

whole that the first picture depicts present progressive ("is washing"), this picture is, by itself, ambiguous between "is washing" and "will wash". Also unclear out of context is the second picture. In general, even with concrete, action verbs, it is hard to depict someone who has not yet performed a particular action but clearly will. Either the future action is not clear or, the more clearly this action is depicted, the more it looks like the actor is already in the act of performing it.

Present progressive, subject-verb agreement, reflexive pronouns, and negated sentences are covered in Laureate's Language Links, but here most of the teaching is incidental, through repeated exposure, rather than explicit. For the most part, the student does not need to attend to the details of the syntactic structure in question to identify the correct picture. As we saw with some of the sentence structure exercises (see Figs. 3.4 and 3.5), the extent to which she learns the syntactic details depends on the extent to which she pays attention.

Additional complex structures are found in Fast ForWord's Language and Ele-bot programs. Both present a number of picture-selection tasks involving prompts with multiple relative clause embeddings, e.g. "The girl that the boy is watching is standing"; "The clown that is holding the balloon that is blue is red";

"The napkin covers the wolf that the basket is holding". Here the teaching and learning are explicit: to determine which picture to click on, the user must sort out which relative clause modifies which noun.

Laureate's QuestionQuest covers one of the most syntactically complex structures of all: namely, questions. This module is particularly comprehensive, requiring the student to discriminate among yes-no questions and the full range of wh-questions. This, at a minimum, requires attention to the specific wh-word used in each question. Figure 3.9 shows one example.

QuestionQuest also covers a type of complex wh-question not seen in the other programs: questions with multiple wh-words, as in "Who is eating what?" and "Who is eating what where?" However, here, while the student may determine the answers by comprehending the question, he could also use a purely pictographic approach, selecting from a picture grid the pairs or triples that match the objects that go together in the larger picture. For example, in Fig. 3.10, it is clear from the picture alone, independently of the syntax and semantics of the question, that the

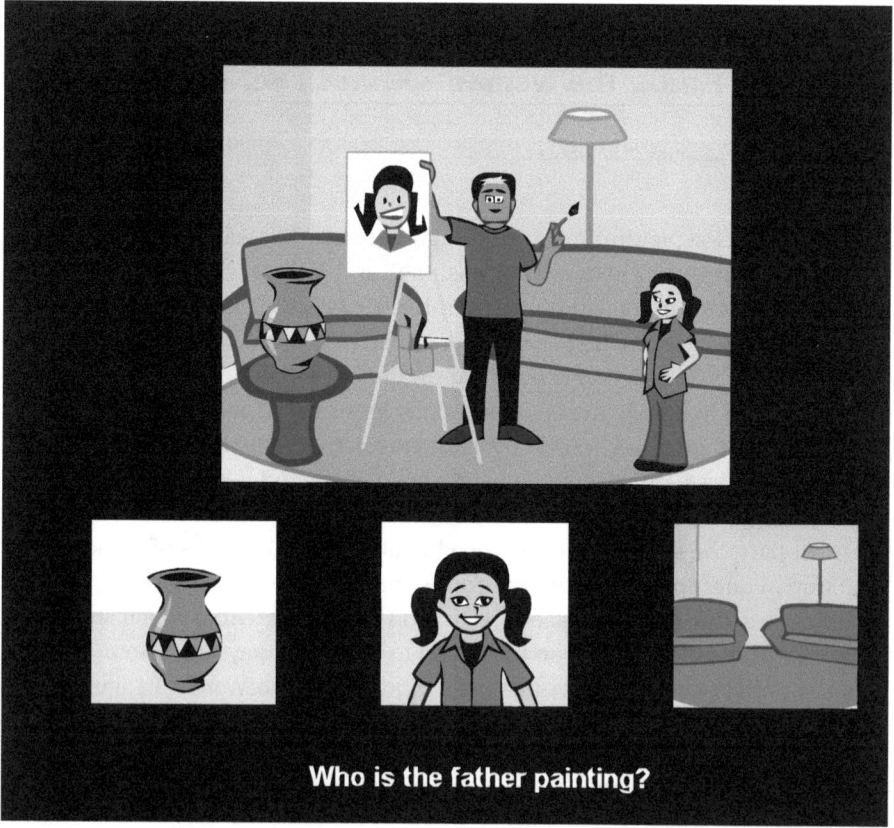

Who is the father painting?

Fig. 3.9: Laureate Learning "QuestionQuest 1".

woman goes with the mug and the light book; the girl, with the dark book and the bottle; and the man, with the newspaper and the large cup.

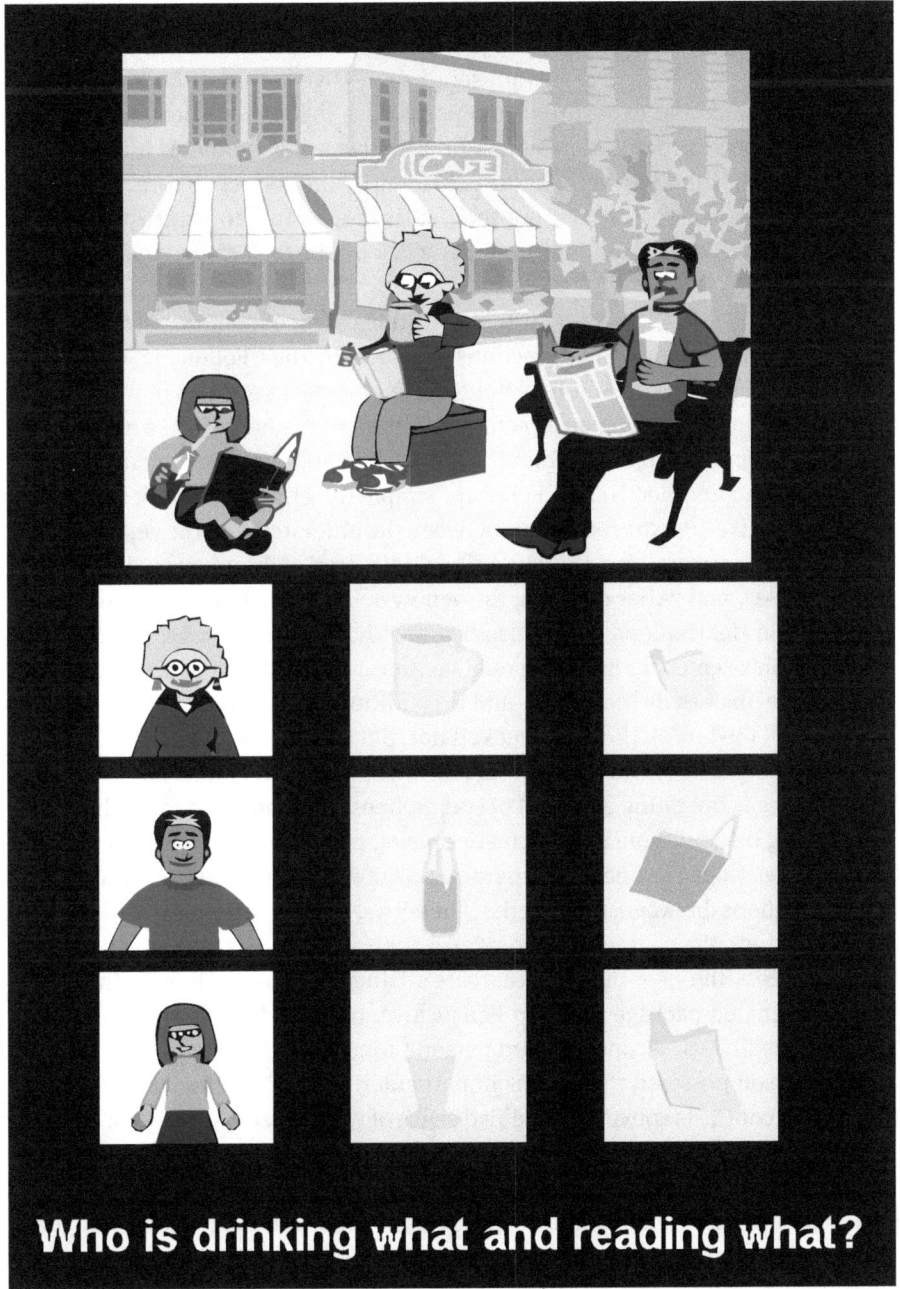

Fig. 3.10: Laureate Learning "QuestionQuest 2".

Another shortcoming of QuestionQuest is that its question prompts are all in the present progressive (e.g. "What is the boy holding"). It therefore does not expose students to the more complex cases of question formation, i.e. those that involve using the appropriate form of "do" and converting the main verb to its bare infinitive form (e.g. "The father paint who" → "Who did the father paint?"). Furthermore, its teaching of this present progressive subset of question syntax is only via incidental exposure: at no point does the student need to attend to the details specific to question syntax (e.g. the overall word order, including the inversion of the auxiliary verb) in order to identify the correct picture. In the case of Fig. 3.9, for example, it is more than sufficient simply to identify the words "who", "father", and "painting" and then click on the only choice that goes with "who": the girl.

Better suited to the explicit teaching and learning of complex sentences are exercises involving complex directions, as seen in the "Following Directions" modules of Fast ForWord and HearBuilder. Here the tasks are also more complex: rather than simply clicking on a picture, the student might click on a sequence of pictures or pictured objects or move around (drag and drop) one pictured object with respect to another. In Fast ForWord, simple directions-following tasks build to sentences like "Put the red square between the blue circle and the yellow circle", "Touch the red square – no, the white circle", "Instead of the green circle touch the yellow circle", and "After touching the yellow square, touch the blue circle". The directions in HearBuilder, which also begin with simple sentences, build to even more complex sentences involving relative clauses – "Click on the large yellow car that is bouncing beside the boat" – and to conditionals such as "If a green doll is in the box, put the box on the large truck; if not, put the box on the small truck". The corresponding tasks, however, are still non-verbal in nature, indicating that linguistic training is operating at a level of comprehension as opposed to production.

Moving beyond syntax to pragmatics, using pictures that show objects nearer to or further from the speaking character, Laureate Learning trains students in the distinctions between the deictics "here" vs. "there" and "this"/"these" vs. "that"/"those". Via characters who address one another or, breaking the "fourth wall", address the user directly, Laureate's Language Links, along with its specially designated package Pronoun Perspective, train students in the distinctions between the first vs. second vs. third person pronouns. When it comes to first and second person possessive pronouns in particular, it should be noted that some of the picture contrasts convey a simplified sense of what possession means: "my cat" is not necessarily the cat that the speaker is holding; "your cat" is not necessarily the cat that the addressee is holding.

What are the strengths and weaknesses of these various receptive language programs? As far as strengths go, certain of the picture-clicking modules show promise in explicitly teaching basic word order (subject-verb-object), basic verb tenses, passive structures, singular vs. plural nouns, wh-words, and what modifies what in sentences with multiple relative clauses. Meanwhile, all of the direction-following modules show promise in explicitly teaching time sequence, conditionals, and relative clause modification. These programs also expose children to many other syntactic patterns in an organized, systematic, repetitive way, in both text-based and oral modalities, thus providing opportunities to learn by implicit exposure.

As for introducing new material, these programs begin by prompting students with the correct answer, and then, consistent with the principles of behaviorist training programs used effectively with children with autism (programs like ABA, or Applied Behavioral Analysis), gradually fade the prompts as the user starts answering correctly. Many of these programs also provide pleasing animated reinforcements for correct answers. Finally, nearly all of them use dynamic algorithms to automatically advance students through the exercises and lessons in accordance with performance. Many, consistent with findings about what constitutes mastery (see, for example, Engelmann 1999), advance students to the next module once they have gotten a certain percentage of trials correct – 80% to 90% is typical. Some instead simply advance students as tasks are completed.

As with the vocabulary programs, the receptive language programs also exploit the ability of software to collect and store user data. Many provide comprehensive reports about different users' levels of mastery of specific modules. As far as speech therapists are concerned, the most useful reports are found in HearBuilder and Laureate, where the modules are described linguistically.

For all the breadth of data, variety of linguistic structures, and systematicity of teaching that these receptive language programs offer, they are dogged by a dearth of randomized controlled studies showing efficacy. Consistent with this are the findings of Bishop, Adams and Rosen (2006). They examine the efficacy of a receptive grammar training program of their own design, used specifically with children with SLI, and focus on distinctions between preposition pairs (e.g. "above" vs. "below") and active and passive sentences. And what they find is that performance improved only for a small number of children, and only on passive constructions.

If the lack of efficacy results reflects an inherent lack of efficacy in these receptive language programs, there are a number of possible contributing factors. First, there is the nature of the feedback provided when answers are wrong. When a user's inputs consist of clicks on pictures, it is hard for the program to diagnose her linguistic errors. This limits the picture selection programs to binary, right-or-wrong feedback – given either by explicitly telling the user that she is right or wrong or, if wrong, by repeating the question and eventually highlighting the correct answer. Recall our earlier discussion of the benefits of elaborative feedback: a lack of meta-linguistic feedback, in particular, limits the user's opportunities to learn from her mistakes.

Then there are the limitations on what can be conveyed through pictures. This constrains grammar instruction as much as it does vocabulary instruction. Pictographic constraints impede, in particular, the instruction of more complex syntax and pragmatics – as discussed above, for example, in the case of possessive pronouns. Consider, as well, the full range of verb forms: tenses other than present tense, aspects other than progressive (e.g. perfective forms like "has finished" and "had finished"), and modes other than indicative and imperative (e.g. the counterfactual "if I were"). Even past tense vs. present tense vs. future tense is quite hard to depict: recall the ambiguity in Fig. 3.8.

Given these limitations on what the comprehension-based, picture-selection programs can and do cover, how well do they potentially prepare language-impaired children for language comprehension in real life? Even if we limit ourselves to those sentences that might plausibly arise in the course of an ordinary day at home or at school, we are talking about thousands of possible sentences. Learning to associate hundreds of canned sentences with corresponding pictures chosen from sets of two to four pre-selected pictures is a far cry from learning to comprehend, within the open-ended context of real life, the thousands of possible everyday sentences of arbitrary length and complexity: anything from "Today we are going to take a look at what happens when we add an odd number to an even number" to "Should we stop off at the store on the way home and pick up some peanut butter and ice cream?" On the other hand, the various receptive training programs may successfully teach crucial first steps, jumpstarting the process of eventually attaining much broader comprehension in open-ended, real-life contexts.

Besides their distance from real-life situations, the contrived environments of these programs have another downside: they make it difficult to guarantee that the child fully comprehends all of a sentence's grammatical details. Perhaps the most extreme example of this we encountered was with QuestionQuest's multiple wh-question exercises. As we saw, these exercises allow the purely pictographic strategy of selecting from the picture grid the pairs or triples that match the objects that go together in the larger picture – as opposed to determining the particular syntactic relationships of the wh-words in the particular questions in which they occur.

How many of the details the user needs to attend to relates to the limitations of receptive language instruction in general. As we discussed earlier in connection with linguistic assessments, often you can comprehend a sentence, even comprehend it fully (i.e. understand it without using key words or picture patterns as crutches), without attending to all the details you would need to learn in order to produce the same sentence. Comprehending questions thoroughly, for example, does not require you to attend to the precise details of do-insertion and subject-auxiliary inversion. Thus, you can understand the question "Who did the father paint" without noticing that it is the auxiliary verb "do", rather than the main verb, that takes the past tense form. Without noticing this, you might, when constructing your own question, erroneously say "Who did the father painted?" or "Who the father painted?" Similarly, you can understand the differences between sentences with singular vs. plural subjects ("The father is painting" vs. "The fathers are painting") without attending to the details of subject-verb agreement. Either you could focus entirely on the subject and the presence or absence of the plural "s" (here, "the father" vs. "the fathers") or you could focus entirely on the verb form (here, "is" vs. "are"). Because you do not need to attend to both the subject and the verb forms together, you can entirely ignore how the one must agree with the other. Thus, a student who understands the difference between "The father is painting" and "The fathers are painting" might still say "The fathers is painting". Similarly, a student might understand the present progressive aspect of "The father is painting" but say "The father painting". Or he might understand possessives like "his coat" but say "he coat", or passives like "The monkey is washed by the monster" but say "The monkey is wash by monster", or relative clause structures like "The clown who is holding the balloon is red" but say "Clown he holding balloon is red".

Consistent with this performance discrepancy, Beals and Hurewitz found in an unpublished study of a GrammarTrainer-based program called QuestionTrainer, the results of which are summarized in Fig. 3.11, that students with autism and grammar difficulties could identify syntactically well-formed questions from a set of choices ("multiple choice responses") at significantly higher rates than they could construct syntactically well-formed questions from scratch ("open-ended responses"). For additional discussion on the different demands of comprehension vs. production, see Clahsen and Felser (2006).

Also at play here may be more general differences between passive and active activities. To what extent can one learn to play the guitar by pure observation – even if what one observes is a series of carefully paced lessons in which all finger movements are clearly indicated? To what extent can one learn to draw a picture of an elephant by watching someone else repeatedly draw a picture of the elephant? To some extent, mastering how to do something requires practice actually doing it. Returning to syntax, or grammar, even in the most ideal of comprehension training environments, there may be substantial limitations on how much grammar a student can master, and, in particular, on the extent to which he or she acquires the ability to actively form the gamut of syntactically correct structures.

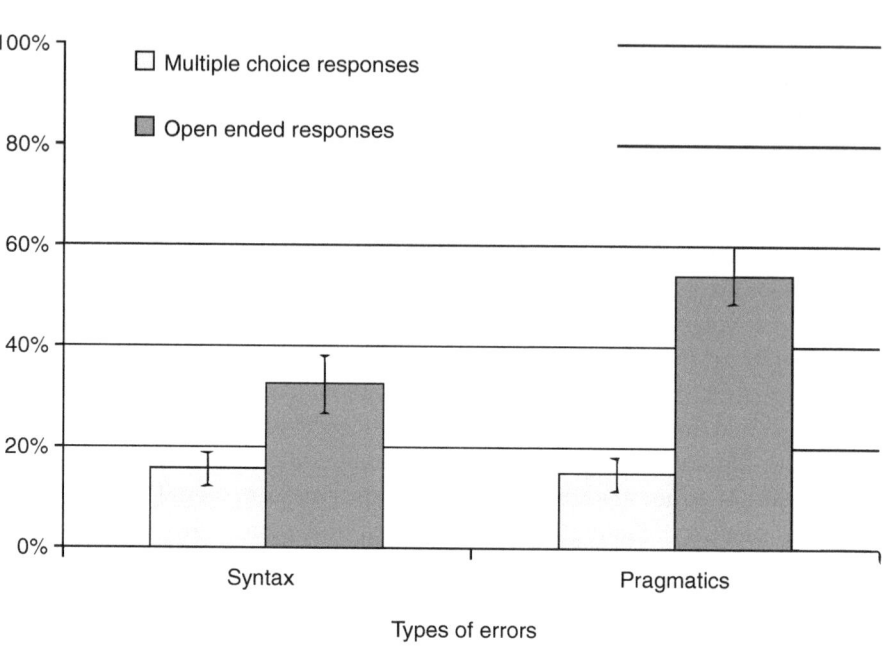

Fig. 3.11: Hurewitz and Beals QuestionTrainer study.

Indeed, research on French language programs for English-speaking students in Quebec highlights the limitations of learning environments that emphasize comprehension over production (Swain 1985). Swain (1985) notes that, in spite of 6 or 7 years of comprehension input in French, the students, who seldom engaged in extended productive language use in class and whose teachers seldom pushed them ahead in their productive skills, made numerous grammatical and syntactic errors in speaking and writing. Swain (1985, 1999) proposes that production prompts listeners to process language more deeply, with more mental effort, and to move "beyond the semantic, open-ended, strategic processing prevalent in comprehension to the complex grammatical processing needed for accurate production". Put another way, the only way to learn to construct phrases is to construct phrases; comprehension practice by itself will not lead to production.

3.2.3 Programs that address productive language

Given that receptive language mastery only gets you so far vis-à-vis full language mastery, any language remediation venture that aspires to bring children to full mastery must include productive language training. Furthermore, as discussed in Chapter 2, a substantial part of the population with autism, along with much of the SLI population, struggles with the types of linguistic features that one can, to some extent, ignore in receptive language training (e.g. the details of verb endings). So we turn now to what exists in the way of productive training programs, beginning with grammar instruction in particular.

In contrast to the picture selection programs that dominate receptive language programs, the productive language programs generally have students selecting words or phrases. One program – NoGlamourGrammar – has students selecting whole sentences. From a choice of just two sentences (e.g. "His shorts are blue" vs. "Him shorts are blue"), students are supposed to click on the one that is grammatically correct. This kind of binary sentence selection task, however, is so far removed from the word-by-word sentence construction that constitutes productive language that we do not dwell on it here. Instead, we focus on the most popular word-selection programs: Laureate's Talking Nouns and Talking Verbs, Mobile Education Store's SentenceBuilder, and Autism Language Therapies' GrammarTrainer.

In the Talking Nouns and Verbs programs, users create short sentences by clicking on sequences of word buttons. Their options, in some sense, are quite open-ended: there are no prompts in these programs that tell users what to say, and so the sentences they construct are entirely at their own initiative. What substantially limits their options, however, is the small number of unchanging word buttons.

Each level of Talking Nouns (there are two in all) provides 25 noun buttons; Talking Verbs provides 40 verb buttons; in all three modules, these buttons display pictures or icons as well as words. In addition, each level contains a set of buttons on the left-hand side with which to begin one's sentences. For Talking Nouns, we find first a column with the pronouns "I", "We", "You", and the phrase "Show me", and then a column with the verbs "see", "want", "have", and "like"; between the two columns at the bottom is the word "do not". This allows the construction of such sentences as "I see boots" and "I do not want eggs". For Talking Verbs, we find a similar selection, except that the verb column contains verbs (or verbal phrases) that can grammatically precede other verbs: "can", "want", "feel like", and "like". This allows such sentences as "I can dance".

In what is called the "sequenced activation" mode, the program speaks aloud the user's input after a phrase or sentence has been constructed, automatically including the correct article or verb form – changing "I want sandwich" to "I want a sandwich" or "I like dance" to "I like dancing". Thus, although users get practice combining root words to form sentences, much of the grammatical work is done for them. Indeed, since there are only root forms for verbs and no buttons for articles, it is in many cases not even possible for users to form grammatical sentences. In addition, the correct sequence of words is strongly hinted at by the left-to-right arrangement of words. Finally, the number of possible permutations is rather small, limiting practice to a small set of very basic sentences.

In SentenceBuilder, the productive language tasks are more varied and grammatically focused – particularly on function words like articles, deictics, and auxiliary verbs. Here, users select words to fill in the blanks of partially constructed sentences that accompany particular pictures. For example, one exercise (see Fig. 3.12) presents a picture of two bears climbing a tree, along with the sentence frame "___ bears ____ climbing ____". The user's choices for the first blank are "the", "then", "that", "this", "it"; for the second, "on", "it", "or", "at", "are"; and for the third, "the ear", "the leaf", "the paw", "the tree", and "the sky". Making the correct selection involves putting the article "the" before the noun "bears" and the auxiliary "are" before the progressive verb "climbing".

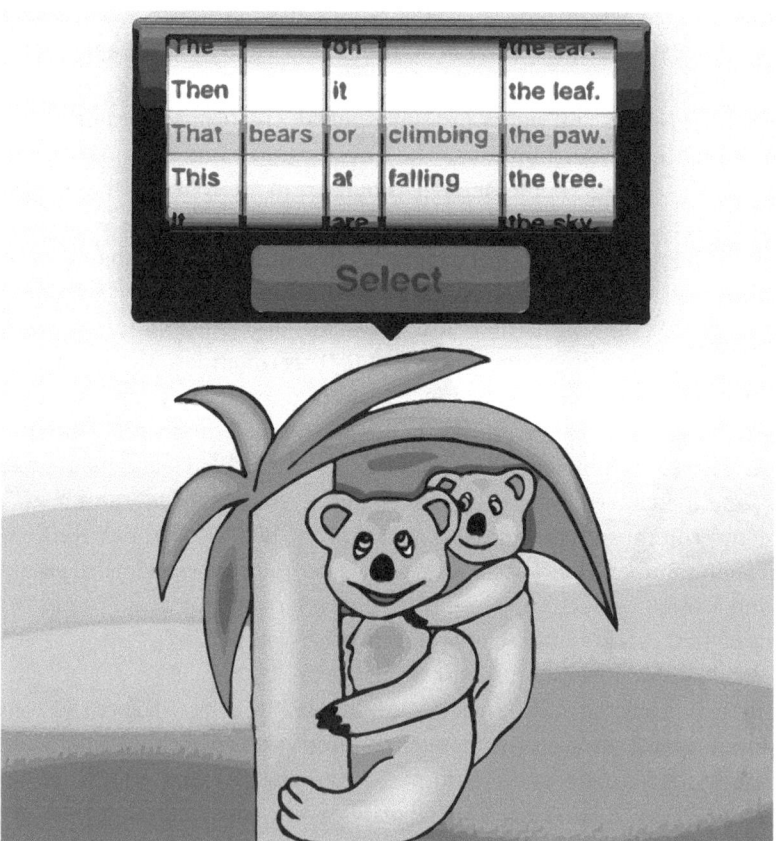

Fig. 3.12: Mobile Education Store SentenceBuilder.

This sort of fill-in-the-blank, word-selection task, however grammatically focused it is, captures only a small subset of the challenges of productive language. For one thing, the syntax and word order are already partially complete when the exercises begin. In the above example, for instance, the subject noun and the two main verb candidates are already positioned, respectively, in the second and fourth slots, and the object noun phrase candidates are already positioned right after the verb. The slot before the subject noun potentially reminds you that you need an article; the slot before the progressive verb reminds you that you need an auxiliary verb. This means that much of the task of remembering to use certain function words and getting the words into the correct order is already completed. Second, there are only a few choices to select among per slot. Both of these factors, in turn, limit SentenceBuilder not just in terms of user input, but in terms of topics covered. In particular, SentenceBuilder does not teach the more complex verb forms and the more challenging aspects of sentence construction.

Thus, neither SentenceBuilder nor Talking Nouns/Verbs trains students in the breadth of productive possibilities that grammar can generate; the unlimited variety of word combinations and sentence structures: "the bears" vs. "some of the bears" vs. "some of the many bears"; "are climbing" vs. "have climbed" vs. "have been climbing" vs. "may have been climbing" – not to mention embedded clauses and other syntactic complexities. Producing an arbitrary sentence, even limiting ourselves to everyday conversation, is a much more open-ended process than selecting words from small sets of fixed buttons or from lists of four to five choices to fill in the blanks of a few hundred sentences that have already been partially constructed for us.

Only a program that actually processes language dynamically is capable of instructing and assisting students in the full range of grammar skills that underlie comprehension and production. The one language teaching program that has these linguistic processing capabilities – and that uses the kind of Natural Language Understanding technology (see Chapter 1 for discussion) necessary for this processing – is GrammarTrainer. Its designer and developer is one of us: a linguist with a background both in grammar and in software development who is also the mother of a boy with autism who turned out to have impairments specifically in grammar. Finding no software program up to the task of teaching her son to speak grammatically, she created her own. And he, from age 6 to 10 years, was GrammarTrainer's first subject – and its beta tester. His progress through the program, of course, counts only as anecdotal data; it resulted, ultimately, in near-complete mastery of all the syntactic structures of English. GrammarTrainer is now under further development as an iPad app known as the SentenceWeaver™.

The key features of the program are the following:

1. A comprehensive, multilevel, multiyear, developmentally sequenced curriculum. This curriculum goes far beyond that covered by other software programs or by traditional therapies. It begins with simple phrases and progresses through increasingly long and complex sentences to cover all the fundamental patterns of English sentences, including the semantics and pragmatics of verb tenses, aspect, and mood (including progressive, perfective, imperative, conditional, counterfactual, and modal), as well as pronouns and a variety of relative clauses, questions, conditionals, and embedded complements.

2. Training in constructing sentences word-by-word from scratch. Users are prompted to construct particular types of sentences that answer particular questions about particular pictures. Users construct sentences by selecting and arranging individual words, selecting them from a set of word buttons that varies from task to task and includes all possible word forms and word choices relevant to the given task. The set of word buttons thus avoids giving away any aspects of the correct answer that pertain to the syntactic features being trained.

3. Interactive feedback that helps the user identify and correct all his/her mistakes. The step-by-step, linguistically informed feedback guides the user, as needed, through a series of corrections to the targeted phrase or sentence, turning user errors into teaching moments and opportunities for active self-correction.

One additional factor that distinguishes GrammarTrainer from other remediation programs is that it requires basic word-recognition skills. It is therefore inaccessible to students who do not read.

Each lesson begins with a teaching phase in which all the choices model grammatically correct versions of the grammatical structure being taught. In the case of the screenshot from Level I, Lesson 7 (Fig. 3.13), the structure in question is "the"+noun+is/are+adjective.

A second phase of the lesson cycles through the same exercises, but with no choices presented, and, to ensure generalization, a third phase of the lesson gives new exercises, again with no choices presented (Fig. 3.14).

The essential ingredient of GrammarTrainer – what enables its unique productive language training – is its complex, linguistically informed Feedback Algorithm. The Feedback Algorithm allows the program to elicit a range of specific productive language targets that include all the fundamental structures of English – structures that span over 100 lessons containing several thousand exercises. For each exercise, for every possible sequence of words that a user might

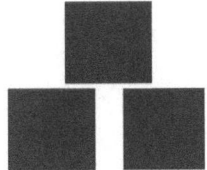

What color are the squares?

CHOICES:
-- The squares are red.
-- The squares are yellow.
-- The squares are blue.
-- The squares are green.

<table><tr><td></td><td>Enter</td><td>Delete</td></tr></table>

Click or type the words to match the correct CHOICE. Then click 'Enter'.

a | an | are | blue | circle | circles | diamond | diamonds | green | is | it | orange | oval | ovals | rectangle | rectangles | red | square | squares | the | them | they | triangle | triangles | yellow

Fig. 3.13: GrammarTrainer Level I Lesson 7 multiple choice.

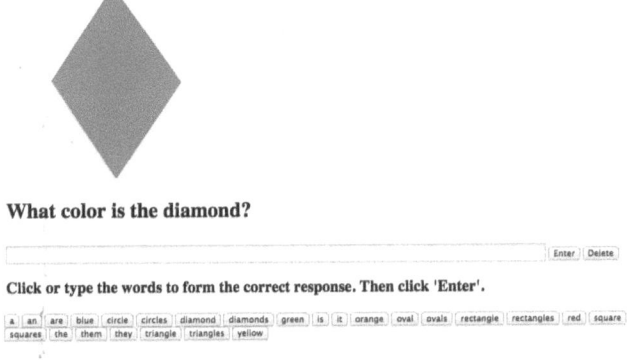

What color is the diamond?

<table><tr><td></td><td>Enter</td><td>Delete</td></tr></table>

Click or type the words to form the correct response. Then click 'Enter'.

a | an | are | blue | circle | circles | diamond | diamonds | green | is | it | orange | oval | ovals | rectangle | rectangles | red | square | squares | the | them | they | triangle | triangles | yellow

Fig. 3.14: GrammarTrainer Lesson 7 open choice.

input, the Feedback Algorithm performs a linguistic analysis and guides the user interactively, step by step, through any necessary revisions – whether in word choice, word endings, word sequencing, or phrase structure – until his or her response is grammatically, semantically, and pragmatically correct.

Fig. 3.15 shows one example of the Feedback Algorithm in action. The student is prompted with a picture of a boy giving a girl a book, along with the question: "What did the boy do to the girl yesterday?" The screens show a series of feedback messages based on the user's errors, which the user corrects one by one on his own.

Saturday, March 28th, 2015 (today it's Sunday, March 29th, 2015):

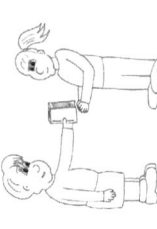

What did the boy do to the girl yesterday?

(Yesterday)

Click or type the words to form the correct response. Then click 'Enter'.

`Enter:` `Delete:`

a | am | are | aren't | book | books | cookie | cookies | cup | cups | did | didn't | do | does | doesn't | doll | don't | gave | get | gets | getting | girls | give | gives | giving | got | he | her | he'll | hers | him | his | is | isn't | it | it's | not | she | she'll | she's | the | their | them | they | they'll | they're | to | will | won't

---

Saturday, March 28th, 2015 (today it's Sunday, March 29th, 2015):

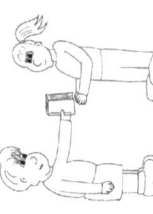

What did the boy do to the girl yesterday?

One word is almost right but has the wrong form. Fix the word in blue.

(Yesterday) he book give to her

(Yesterday) he book give to her

Click or type the words to form the correct response. Then click 'Enter'.

`Enter:` `Delete:`

a | am | are | aren't | book | books | cookie | cookies | cup | cups | did | didn't | do | does | doesn't | doll | don't | gave | get | gets | getting | girls | give | gives | giving | got | he | her | he'll | hers | him | his | is | isn't | it | it's | not | she | she'll | she's | the | their | them | they | they'll | they're | to | will | won't

---

Saturday, March 28th, 2015 (today it's Sunday, March 29th, 2015):

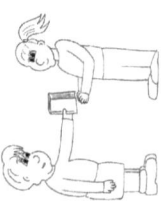

What did the boy do to the girl yesterday?

You need the word book. Please type it in.

(Yesterday) he give to her

Click or type the words to form the correct response. Then click 'Enter'.

`Enter:` `Delete:`

a | am | are | aren't | book | books | cookie | cookies | cup | cups | did | didn't | do | does | doesn't | doll | don't | gave | get | gets | getting | girls | give | gives | giving | got | he | her | he'll | hers | him | his | is | isn't | it | it's | not | she | she'll | she's | the | their | them | they | they'll | they're | to | will | won't

---

Saturday, March 28th, 2015 (today it's Sunday, March 29th, 2015):

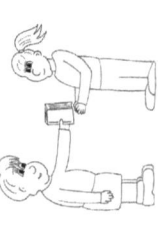

What did the boy do to the girl yesterday?

One word has the wrong ending. Change or delete the ending in red.

(Yesterday) he book gaved to her

(Yesterday) he book gaved to her

Click or type the words to form the correct response. Then click 'Enter'.

`Enter:` `Delete:`

a | am | are | aren't | book | books | cookie | cookies | cup | cups | did | didn't | do | does | doesn't | doll | don't | gave | get | gets | getting | girls | give | gives | giving | got | he | her | he'll | hers | him | his | is | isn't | it | it's | not | she | she'll | she's | the | their | them | they | they'll | they're | to | will | won't

Saturday, March 28th, 2015 (today it's Sunday, March 29th, 2015):

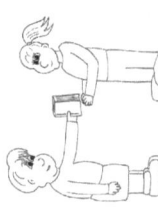

What did the boy do to the girl yesterday?

The word in blue needs an article. Please type a, an, or the in the correct space.

(Yesterday) he book gave to her

(Yesterday) he book gave to her

Click or type the words to form the correct response. Then click 'Enter'.

[a | an | aren't | book | books | cookie | cookies | cup | cups | did | didn't | do | does | doesn't | doll | don't | gave | get | gets | getting | girls | give | gives | giving | got | he | her | he'll | hers | him | his | is | isn't | it | it's | not | she | she'll | she's | the | their | them | they | they'll | they're | to | will | won't]   Enter Delete

Saturday, March 28th, 2015 (today it's Sunday, March 29th, 2015):

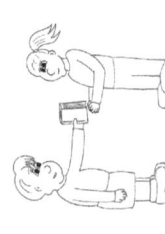

What did the boy do to the girl yesterday?

Some of your words are in the wrong order (1st, 2nd, 3rd,...). Change the order of the words in red.

(Yesterday) he a book gave to her

(Yesterday) he a book gave to her

Click or type the words to form the correct response. Then click 'Enter'.

[a | an | aren't | book | books | cookie | cookies | cup | cups | did | didn't | do | does | doesn't | doll | don't | gave | get | gets | getting | girls | give | gives | giving | got | he | her | he'll | hers | him | his | is | isn't | it | it's | not | she | she'll | she's | the | their | them | they | they'll | they're | to | will | won't]   Enter Delete

Saturday, March 28th, 2015 (today it's Sunday, March 29th, 2015):

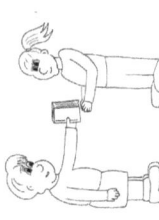

What did the boy do to the girl yesterday?

(Yesterday) he gave a book to her

Click or type the words to form the correct response. Then click 'Enter'.

[a | an | aren't | book | books | cookie | cookies | cup | cups | did | didn't | do | does | doesn't | doll | don't | gave | get | gets | getting | girls | give | gives | giving | got | he | her | he'll | hers | him | his | is | isn't | it | it's | not | she | she'll | she's | the | their | them | they | they'll | they're | to | will | won't]   Enter Delete

Good job! That's right.

Fig. 3.15: (a–g) GrammarTrainer Level II Lesson 27.

When the user fixes the final error, putting "a book gave" in the correct order to yield "He gave her a book", the program congratulates him and moves on to the next exercise.

The feedback is fairly elaborative, particularly in the verbal explanation of what is wrong. But what draws the eye is the colored text beneath, (which appears here as grayed-out text), and this, essentially, boils down to right-or-wrong feedback. The words highlighted in red and blue are the ones that, in some sense, are wrong, and one can attend merely to them and still make appropriate corrections. Supporting this combination of elaborative and right-or-wrong feedback are our observations earlier in the chapter about which factors appear to optimize learning, particularly in the case of grammar.

Recall, now, our earlier discussion of grammar assessments. We saw there how difficult it is for traditional tests with human examiners to elicit some of the more complex syntactic structures – for example, complex verb tenses, questions, and sentences with embedded clauses. GrammarTrainer's picture sequencing, rigid format, and the specific limitations it imposes on the user (providing only certain word buttons; requiring the user to use certain words) is better poised to elicit these structures. Figure 3.16 shows how GrammarTrainer elicits future perfect tense.

Figure 3.17 shows how GrammarTrainer teaches and elicits abstract time prepositions, in this case, "until".

In these and other exercises, GrammarTrainer, via temporal phrases like "now", "yesterday", and "in two minutes", bypasses the earlier-discussed limits on how well pictures convey verb tense. Making this possible, in part, are earlier

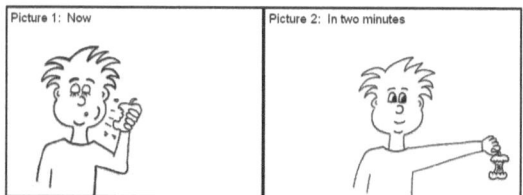

Complete the sentence about Picture 2, WITHOUT using the word FINISH.
In two minutes...

Click or type the words to form the correct response. Then click 'Enter'.

Fig. 3.16: GrammarTrainer Level III Lesson 24.

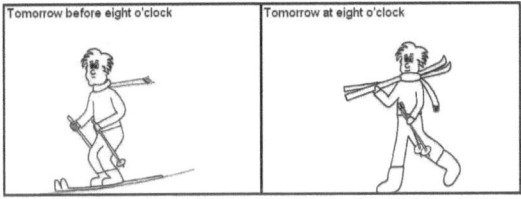

How long will the boy ski?

Click or type the words to form the correct response. Then click 'Enter'.

Fig. 3.17: GrammarTrainer Level III Lesson 25.

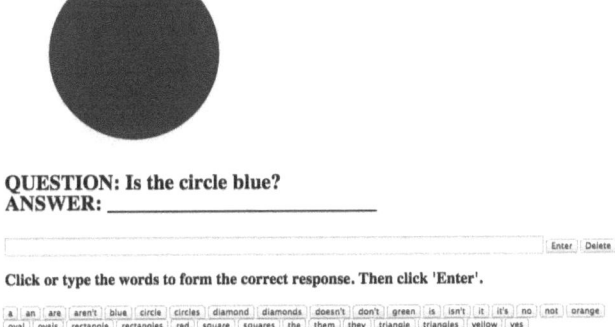

Click or type the words to form the correct response. Then click 'Enter'.

Fig. 3.18: GrammarTrainer Level I Lesson 24.

lessons that use the computer's internal clock to teach the gamut of basic time expressions.

As for teaching and eliciting questions, first GrammarTrainer presents a series of exercises that model the question, label it as a "question", and place it right above a blank line labeled "answer" (see Fig. 3.18). As the user constructs the response, the words (or word) then appear in the answer field.

Next, it shows a series of counterparts in which the "question" field is blank and the "answer" field is full. As in the quiz show Jeopardy, the user's job is now to construct the question that goes with the answer, in this case, "Is the circle blue?" (Fig. 3.19).

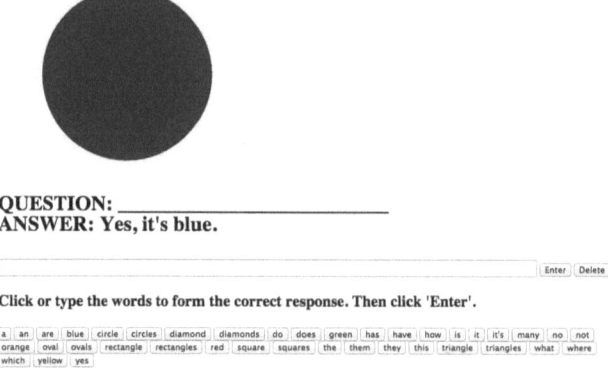

QUESTION: _____
ANSWER: Yes, it's blue.

Click or type the words to form the correct response. Then click 'Enter'.

a | an | are | blue | circle | circles | diamond | diamonds | do | does | green | has | have | how | is | it | it's | many | no | not | orange | oval | ovals | rectangle | rectangles | red | square | squares | the | them | they | this | triangle | triangles | what | where | which | yellow | yes

Fig. 3.19: GrammarTrainer Level I Lesson 24.

<u>**Yesterday (Saturday, March 28th, 2015):**</u>

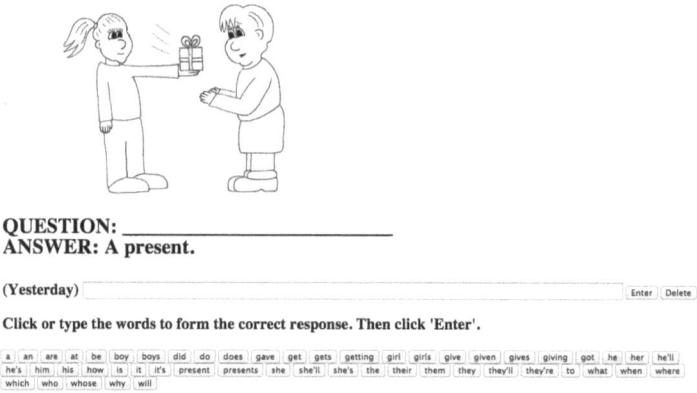

QUESTION: _____
ANSWER: A present.

(Yesterday)

Click or type the words to form the correct response. Then click 'Enter'.

a | an | are | at | be | boy | boys | did | do | does | gave | get | gets | getting | girl | girls | give | given | gives | giving | got | he | her | he'll | he's | him | his | how | is | it | it's | present | presents | she | she'll | she's | the | their | them | they | they'll | they're | to | what | when | where | which | who | whose | why | will

Fig. 3.20: GrammarTrainer Level III Lesson 11.

Later, the program moves on to wh-questions ("What did the girl give to the boy?") (Fig. 3.20).

In the course of these question-and-answer exercises, the user learns, not just the syntax of questions (including the do-insertion and subject-auxiliary inversion that elude so many assessments and training programs) but also their rudimentary pragmatics: the question is the thing that goes right before the answer.

In not letting the user submit her answer until she uses certain words, the program can elicit certain very specific structures. In the example in Fig. 3.21,

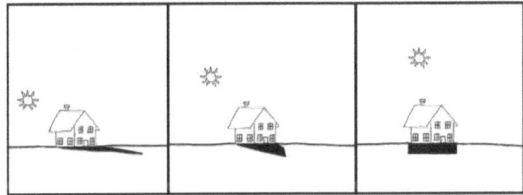

Describe the picture, using the words:
DEPEND, SUN, HIGH, SHADOW, SHORT.

(Any day) How short the shadow is depends on how high the sun is.   Enter Delete

Click or type the words to form the correct response. Then click 'Enter'.

a | an | are | be | depend | depended | depending | depends | did | do | does | he | her | he'll | he's | high | him | his | how | is | it | it's | late
long | low | moon | on | shadow | she | she'll | she's | short | sun | tall | the | their | them | they | they'll | they're | will

Fig. 3.21: GrammarTrainer Level III Lesson 23.

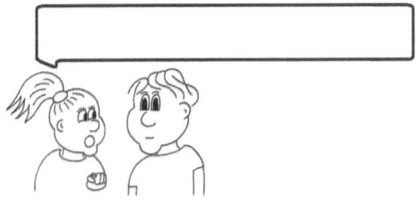

The girl said that she wants you to watch her.
What did the girl say? (Don't use the words SAID THAT).

                                                                         Enter Delete

Click or type the words to form the correct response. Then click 'Enter'.

a | an | are | boy | boys | did | do | does | girl | girls | he | her | herself | he'd | he'll | he's | him | himself | his | I | is | it | I'd
I'll | I'm | left | left's | me | my | myself | our | right | right's | said | say | saying | she | she'd | she'll | she's | the | their | them
themselves | they | they'd | they'll | they're | to | us | want | wanted | wanting | wants | watch | watched | watches | watching | we
we'd | we'll | we're | will | would | you | your | yourself | yourselves | you'd | you'll | you're

Fig. 3.22: GrammarTrainer Level IV Lesson 1.

we see the elicitation of a particular comparative structure involving the clausal subject "How short the shadow is".

In our discussion of traditional language therapies, we saw how difficult it is to teach the pronoun distinctions with which many children with autism struggle: "I"/"me" vs. "you" vs. "he"/"she". GrammarTrainer does this via exercises that have students translate reported speech ("The girl says that she wants you to watch her") into direct speech ("You need to watch me") based on who the characters are speaking to and referring to, with cartoon balloons that fill up with the words the user clicks into the response box. One example from Level IV is shown in Fig. 3.22.

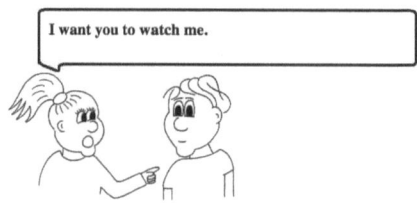

What did the girl say? (Use the words SAY and THAT).

| | Enter | Delete |

Click or type the words to form the correct response. Then click 'Enter'.

a · an · are · boy · boys · did · do · does · girl · girls · he · her · herself · he'd · he'll · he's · him · himself · his · I · is · it · I'd

Fig. 3.23: GrammarTrainer Level IV Lesson 2.

A set of parallel exercises have the user change direct speech into reported speech (Fig. 3.23).

Collectively, the dozens of exercises in this module present, in randomized order, every possible combination of the variables that determine pronoun use: where the speaker is looking, where he is pointing, and what he is directly or reportedly saying. Sometimes, the speaker points to and looks at the user; sometimes, she points to and looks at the other character; and sometimes, she points to one person and looks at the other. The feedback the user receives if his pronoun choice is wrong avoids the pitfalls of the in-person, face-to-face corrections we discussed earlier in this chapter: just as it does with incorrect word choices in general, the program simply highlights the wrong word in red and identifies it as "wrong or extra". This, combined with the systematicity and intensity of instruction, provides the kind of rigorous training in pronoun use to which in-person therapy is far less conducive.

In learning to choose situationally appropriate pronouns, as well as learning, in earlier lessons, to form situationally appropriate questions, students acquire, not just productive grammar, but also certain specific elements of productive pragmatics. Furthermore, in the course of the Level IV pronoun exercises, the student not only practices making pronoun distinctions, but also works with a type of embedded clause structure that turns out to be particularly significant vis-à-vis other deficits in autism, as we will discuss below.

Two pedagogical principles guide the strategies used by GrammarTrainer. One is the notion that to fully master the syntactic elements of language, children need to learn them in a developmentally appropriate sequence. Consistent with this, it teaches auxiliary verbs as used in negation ("The boy did not wave to the girl") before teaching the question patterns that also use such auxiliary verbs, but in a more complex way ("Did the boy wave to the girl?"). This is supported by Krashen's "natural order of acquisition" hypothesis (Krashen 1982; Thomke & Boser 2011).

Another guiding principle, of course, is the above-discussed value of productive practice: the principle that to fully master such sentence formation skills, children need to practice them actively, by selecting words and constructing sentences.

What then is known of the actual efficacy of GrammarTrainer? As with most of the commercially available grammar programs we have surveyed here, including the other productive language programs (Talking Nouns/Verbs and SentenceBuilder), there are, to date, no published, randomized controlled studies. However, three preliminary unpublished pilot studies indicate promise. Two of these are of the basic lessons in phrase formation (from Level I); the third is of the intermediate lessons in question formation (from Level II). All three studies show improvements from pretest to posttest, including (in one study) improvements on the syntax subtest of the CASL even after just 3 weeks of training (see Dressler 2011). Methodological flaws make these studies far from definitive; their promising results, however, call out for additional studies.

Given the size of the curriculum, the ideal study would include a large number of subjects, a placement test that starts different students at different points in the curriculum, and a training protocol that lasts many months. Improvements in grammar should be measured by independent, standardized tests like those discussed in Section 3.1, with particular attention paid to how improvements in the grammar-based tests or subtests compare with improvements in other areas of language.

Beyond grammar, there is one particular skill worth measuring, even though it is neither something directly trained by the program nor even linguistic in nature. The skill in question is the ability to reason about false beliefs, as manifested, for example, in an experiment known as the "Sally-Anne Experiment". This experiment involves two puppets, Sally and Anne, as well as a marble, a box, and a basket. While Sally is watching, Anne puts the marble in the box. Sally leaves the room, and while she is gone, Anne moves the marble from the basket to the box. Sally returns, and subjects are asked: "Where will Sally look for the marble?" Reasoning through to the correct answer, "in the basket", involves reasoning about false beliefs – namely, Sally's false belief about where the marble is. Children younger than 3 years generally answer incorrectly ("in the box"); children with autism continue to do so long after typically developing children start answering correctly. As it turns out (see de Villiers & de Villiers 2003), the ability to reason about false beliefs is correlated with the mastery of a particular syntactic structure, namely, the sentential complements of certain verbs. These are the embedded clauses found in such sentences as "Sally thinks that the marble is in the basket" or "Sally said that the marble is in the basket", where the proposition expressed by the embedded clause ("the marble is in the basket") can be false at the same time that the proposition expressed by the entire sentence ("Sally thinks/says that the marble is in the basket") is true.

Studies (see de Villiers & de Villiers 2003) have found that the subpopulation with autism is not the only group that struggles with the Sally-Anne test. A subpopulation of deaf children is also delayed in passing false belief tests: namely, those children whose exposure to language (whether spoken language or signed language) is limited or delayed and who therefore are delayed in acquiring the syntax of embedded complements. Additional research suggests a particular direction of causality: training in embedded clause syntax improves performance on the Sally-Anne and other false belief tests (rather than vice versa). Since one of the many syntactic structures trained by GrammarTrainer are the embedded complements of Level IV (see Fig. 3.22 and Fig 3.23), one could test whether training here leads to improvements in false belief tests. One could also explore whether any other GrammarTrainer modules foster such improvements. One candidate is a module in Level III in which the distinctions among first, second, and third person pronouns are first taught. To make these distinctions, as we have discussed, one must learn to take different perspectives. Taking different perspectives, in turn, might be another mechanism for calculating variations in what different people believe.

Besides better and more comprehensive efficacy testing, what else would improve GrammarTrainer – or any program that aspires to teach productive grammar? One is better picture prompts, particularly in those exercises, like pronoun exercises, in which the eye contact and pointing gestures comprise part of the visual prompt. Animation of gestures and eye gaze would also make these prompts clearer and more reflective of the real-world cues that guide real-world communication. In fact, the SentenceWeaver, the iPad version of GrammarTrainer currently under development, has both improved the pictures and added animation – for precisely these purposes.

GrammarTrainer could also use more user-friendly word buttons. Indeed, well-organized, user friendly word buttons are essential in any productive language teaching program that aspires to cover all the challenges of productive grammar. As seen in the above screenshots of GrammarTrainer, some of the exercises, in order not to give away the correct answers, present rather long lists of buttons. Currently organized alphabetically, they might be easier to navigate if also grouped according to part of speech, with different part-of-speech buttons bringing up different word buttons. That is currently the design being tested in SentenceWeaver. GrammarTrainer does allow users to enter their answers by typing, but this is faster only for those whose keyboarding skills are fairly advanced.

GrammarTrainer could also use better data collection. Currently, the only data collected is temporary, within-session data. The SentenceWeaver, on the other hand, records all user inputs, including incremental responses to feedback, and is thus poised to process a great deal of information about student learning and progress.

One limitation seen in all the linguistic software programs for autism and SLI is that none of them teach productive speech. Even the few that teach productive grammar, like GrammarTrainer, have students submitting text rather than simply speaking. But evidence from syntactic priming experiments suggests that spoken and written language production involve the same underlying syntactic and semantic processes (Cleland & Pickering 2006). If so, then the improvements in written production targeted by programs like GrammarTrainer will generalize to spoken language.

On the other hand, as with Fast ForWord above, adding a speech recognizer could make training more robust. In this case, the speech recognizer could use a speech recognition grammar (see Chapter 1 for discussion) that limits the input it recognizes to that which can be generated from GrammarTainer's word buttons – substantially increasing its potential efficacy. It would then convert oral responses into text messages both for the Feedback Algorithm and to display in the answer fields. Add in a TTS component that reads out the written prompts and the wrong-answer feedback, and the program becomes at least somewhat accessible to nonreaders – as well as considerably more user-friendly to everyone. Speaking a phrase or sentence is significantly faster than typing it, let alone searching for appropriate word buttons and selecting them one at a time.

The problem, again, is that the speech recognizer would have to be extremely sophisticated: both forgiving enough to capture the often imperfectly articulated phonemes of child speech, particularly the speech of children with language impairments, while remaining unforgiving of syntactic errors, many of which (for example, morphological endings like -s and -ed) may involve only subtle acoustic distinctions. In other words, the recognizer would need to recognize both poorly articulated words and syntactic errors that may also be poorly articulated. It would need to recognize them well enough to distinguish between the two and well enough to provide accurate transcriptions of the syntax errors to the Feedback Algorithm. On the other hand, imperfect speech recognition might still provide some benefits: those children who are able to read the speech recognizer output could at least see that the recognizer was wrong and try again.

Are there additional aspects of grammar or pragmatics that a productive language software program might teach? As discussed, GrammarTrainer covers all the fundamental syntactic structures of English. In terms of pragmatics, as we have seen, it covers first, second, and third person pronoun distinctions, and as seen in the discussion of its question elicitation methodology, in which it pairs particular questions with corresponding answers, it also covers the basic pragmatics of what a question is for. However, there are some regular, context-free pragmatics rules suitable to computerized training that GrammarTrainer does not cover: namely deictics like "this" vs. "that" and "here" vs. "there". These involve the same kinds of perspective taking as pronouns do: "here" and "this" are used in reference to areas and objects near the speaker; "there" and "that" for areas and objects away from the speaker. The same sort of format involving pointing characters and cartoon balloons used to teach pronouns could also be used to teach deictics.

A more challenging aspect of pragmatics is the distinction between the indefinite and definite articles "a" and "the". Fully articulating the rules for when to use the definite ("the") vs. the indefinite ("a") has eluded even linguists – particularly those involved in teaching this distinction to second-language learners whose first languages do not make this distinction (see Master 2002). However, some of the distinctions between "a" and "the" are relatively straightforward. If there is more than one cookie present and we do not care which one we get, we say, "Can you give me a cookie?" If there's only one cookie we say, "Can you give me the cookie?" If we want a particular cookie among several present, we say "the" but add distinguishing features: "Can you give me the cookie with the green frosting?" A series of GrammarTrainer-type exercises could capture at least these basic patterns.

As discussed earlier, however, the more the vicissitudes of the real world figure into pragmatic distinctions, the harder it is for linguistic software to capture and teach them. And the more open-ended the range of pragmatically felicitous responses is, the harder these responses are to assess.

There is, however, the potential, discussed earlier, of dialog systems and apps like Siri to give students safe, pressure-free ways to practice their conversational skills. Along these lines, specifically intended for people with weaknesses in conversational skills, is Simmersion. Simmersion attempts to teach these skills in a real-world simulation via an actual human "conversational partner". The way this works is that clips of this partner are pre-recorded, and the user has to select among several pre-packaged conversational responses. For example, when asked, "Are you into computers?", the user chooses among "Not really", "No, I think they are boring", "Yes", and "Yeah, I spend a lot of time on my home computer". Depending on whether his choice is more conversationally felicitous ("Not really" or "Yeah, I spend a lot of time on my home computer") or less so ("No, I think they are boring", "Yes"), other pre-recorded clips in the lower right corner of the screen show a human "observer" expressing either approval or dismay.

Obviously, this does not come close to simulating the realities of open-ended conversation, with its lack of canned responses to choose from and its infinite variety of real-life contexts. Nonetheless, a program like Simmersion may serve as a starting point in helping pragmatically impaired individuals with autism consider issues of pragmatic appropriateness. A recent efficacy study of a module of Simmersion that specifically simulates job interviews finds that users improved their performance relative to control subjects in live, standardized, job interview role-playing activities (Smith et al. 2014). Efficacy studies on broader conversational skills training via Simmersion have yet to be published.

The same is true, as we have seen, of studies on the efficacy of the grammar training programs. However, given the abstract, rule-based essence of grammar vs. the open-endedness and real-world entanglements of pragmatics, it is worth concluding this section by recapping the point that, while most grammar deficits are potentially remediable by linguistic software programs, most pragmatic deficits are not.

A second concluding remark is also in order: when it comes to computerized training in spoken language, effective speech recognition technology is essential, and the requisite efficacy probably requires some significant advancements beyond current technology.

References

Bishop, D. V., Adams, C. V. & Rosen, S. (2006). Resistance of grammatical impairment to computerized comprehension training in children with specific and non-specific language impairments. *International Journal of Language and Communication Disorders 41*, 19–40.

Bloom, P. (2002). Mindreading, communication, and learning the names for things. *Mind & Language, 17*, 37–54.

Bosseler, A. & Massaro, D. (2003). Development and evaluation of a computer-animated tutor for vocabulary and language learning in children with autism. *Journal of Autism and Developmental Disorders 33*, 653–672.

Cassady, J. C., Smith, L. L. & Linda, K. (2005). Enhancing validity in phonological awareness assessment through computer-supported testing. *Practical Assessment, Research And Evaluation, 10*. Retrieved from http://pareonline.net/getvn.asp?v=10&n=18

Chen, S. H. A. & Bernard-Opitz, V. (1993). Comparison of personal and computerized instruction for children with autism. *Mental Retardation 31*, 368–376.

Clahsen, H. & Felser, C. (2006). Grammatical processing in language learners. *Applied Psycholinguistics, 27*, 3–42.

Cleland, A. & Pickering, M. (2006). Do writing and speaking employ the same syntactic representations? *Journal of Memory and Language, 54*, 185–198.

de Villiers, J. G. & de Villiers, P. A. (2003). Language for thought: Coming to understand false beliefs. In D. Gentner & S. Goldin-Meadow (Eds.), *Language in Mind: Advances in the Study of Language and Thought* (pp. 335–384). Cambridge, MA: MIT Press.

Dressler, J. (2011). *The generalization of text-based computer-aided instruction to verbal speech production by students with autism.* Philadelphia, PA: Drexel University.

Engelmann, S. (1999). Student-program alignment and teaching to mastery. In *25th National Direct Instruction Conference.*

Freeman, S. & Dake, L. (1997). *Teach Me language: A language manual for children with autism, Asperger's syndrome and related developmental disorders.* Langley, BC, Canada: SKF Books.

Greenspan, S. I. & Lewis, D. (2005). *The affect-based language curriculum (ABLC),* 2nd ed. Exeter, UK: Revaluation Books.

Happé, F. G. E. (1995). Understanding minds and metaphors: Insights from the study of figurative language in autism. *Metaphor and Symbolic Activity, 10,* 275–295.

Heim, S., Keil, A., Choudhury, N., Thomas Friedman, J. & Benasich, A. (2013). Early gamma oscillations during rapid auditory processing in children with a language-learning impairment: Changes in neural mass activity after training. *Neuropschologia, 51,* 990–1001.

Heimann, M., Nelson, K., Tjus, T. & Gillberg, C. (1995). Increasing reading and communication skills in children with autism through an interactive multimedia program. *Journal of Autism and Developmental Disorders 25,* 459–480.

Hewitt, L. E., Hammer, C. S., Yont, K. M. & Tomblin, J. B. (2005). Language sampling for kindergarten children with and without SLI: Mean length of utterance, IPSYN, and NDW. *Journal of Communication Disorders, 38,* 197–213.

Hurewitz, F. & Beals, K. (2008). Role for grammar in autism CAIs. In *IDC '08 Proceedings of the 7th International Conference on Interaction Design and Children* (pp. 73–76). New York: ACM.

Krashen, S. (1982). *Principles and practice in second language acquisition.* Oxford: Pergamon Press.

Kulik, C. -L., Kulik, J. A. & Bangert-Drowns, R. L. (1990). Effectiveness of mastery learning programs: A meta-analysis. *Review of Educational Research, 60,* 265–299.

Lavie, A., MacWhinney, B. & Sagae, K. (2005). *Automatic measurement of syntactic development in child language.* Carnegie Mellon University, Department of Psychology, Dietrich College of Humanities and Social Sciences.

Long, S. H., Fey, M. E. & Channell, R. W. (2004). *Computerized profiling (Version 9.6.0).* Cleveland, OH: Case Western Reserve University.

Mason, B. J. & Bruning, R. (2001). *Providing feedback in computer-based instruction: What the research tells us.* Retrieved from http://dwb.unl.edu/Edit/MB/MasonBruning.html

Master, P. (2002). Information structure and English article pedagogy. *System, 30,* 331–348.

Moore, M. & Calvert, S. (2000). Brief report: Vocabulary acquisition for children with autism: Teacher or computer instruction. *Journal of Autism and Developmental Disorders, 30,* 359–360.

Newman, J. (2014, October 17). To Siri, with love: How one boy with autism became BFF with Apple's Siri. *New York Times.* Retrieved from http://www.nytimes.com/2014/10/19/fashion/how-apples-siri-became-one-autistic-boys-bff.html?r=1

Palyu, W. (n.d.). *Grateful grammar! Fall/Thanksgiving themed grammar unit.* Retrieved from http://www.teacherspayteachers.com/Product/Grateful-Grammar-FallThanksgiving-Themed-Grammar-Unit-946210

Pridemore, D. R. & Klein, J. D. (1991). Control of feedback in computer-assisted instruction. *Educational Technology Research and Development, 39,* 27–32.

Rogowsky, B. A., Papamichalis, P., Villa, L., Heim, S. & Tallal, P. (2013). Neuroplasticity-based cognitive and linguistic skills training improves reading and writing skills in college students. *Frontiers in Psychology, 4,* 137.

Roper, W. J. (1977). Feedback in computer assisted instruction. *Programmed Learning and Educational Technology, 14,* 43–49.

Scarborough, H. S. (1990). Index of productive syntax. *Applied Psycholinguistics, 11,* 1–22.

Simmersion. http://www.simmersion.com/

Smith, J. D., Boomer, J., Zakrzewski, A. C., Roeder, J. L., Church, B. A. & Ashby, F. G. (2013). Deferred feedback sharply dissociates implicit and explicit category learning. *Psychological Science, 25,* 447.

Smith M. J., Ginger E. M., Wright K., Wright M. A., Taylor J. L., Boteler H. L., Olsen D., Bell M. B., Fleming M. F. (2014). Virtual reality job interview training in adults with autism spectrum disorder. *Journal of Autism and Developmental Disorders, 44,* 2450–2463.

Stanovich, K. E., Cunningham, A. E. & Cramer, B. B. (1984). Assessing phonological awareness in kindergarten children: Issues of task comparability. *Journal of Experimental Child Psychology, 38,* 175–190.

Strong, G. K., Torgerson, C. J., Torgerson, D. & Hulme, C. (2011). A systematic meta-analytic review of evidence for the effectiveness of the 'Fast ForWord' language intervention program. *Child Psychology and Psychiatry, 52,* 224–235.

Swain, M. (1985). Communicative competence: Some roles of comprehensible input and comprehensible output in its development. In S. Gass & C. Madden (Eds.). *Input in second language acquisition* 235–253. Rowley, MA: Newbury House.

Swain, M. (1999). French immersion research in Canada: Recent contributions to SLA and applied linguistics. *Annual Review of Applied Linguistics, 12,* 199–212.

Thomke, H. & Boser, K. (2011). Language construction in an autistic child: Thoughts regarding language acquisition and language therapy: Translation, update, and commentary on a 1977 case report. *Cognitive and Behavioral Neurology, 24,* 156–156.

Ullman, M., Corkin, S., Coppola, M., Hickok, G., Growdon, J. H., Koroshetz, W. J., Pinker, S. (1997). Neural dissociation within language: Evidence that the mental dictionary is part of declarative memory, and that grammatical rules are processed by the procedural system. *Journal of Cognitive Neuroscience, 9,* 266–276.

Waldrop, P. B., Justen, J. E. & Adams, T. M. (1986). A comparison of three types of feedback in a computer-assisted instruction task. *Educational Technology, 26,* 43–45.

Whalen, C., Moss, D., Ilan, A. B., Vaupel, M., Fielding, P., Macdonald, K., Cernich, S., Symon, J. (2010). Efficacy of TeachTown: Basics computer-assisted intervention for the intensive comprehensive autism program in Los Angeles unified school district. *Autism: International Journal of Research and Practice, 14,* 179–197.

Whyte, M. M., Karolick, D. M., Neilsen, M. C., Elder, G. D. & Hawley, W. T. (1995). Cognitive styles and feedback in computer-assisted instruction. *Journal of Educational Computing Research, 12,* 195–203.

Xin, Y. P. & Jitendra, A. K. (1999). The effects of instruction in solving mathematical word problems for students with learning problems: A meta-analysis. *Journal of Special Education, 32,* 207–225.

Katharine Beals

4 Technology for task assessment, classroom accommodation, and communicative assistance of developmental language disorders

Abstract: This chapter discusses potential and existing technologies for assisting language-impaired students in classrooms. It begins with technologies that assess linguistic challenges, particularly those found in reading assignments. Next it discusses accommodations, particularly TTS, speech-to-text, and text simplification software. Finally, it surveys devices that assist with in-person communication and written assignments.

The prospects of language-impaired children, as of all children, depend largely on their successful advancement through school. Here, a huge amount of instruction occurs through written and oral language, and a huge proportion of tasks involve reading and writing. The academic success and real-life prospects of children with language impairments thus depend largely on the extent to which the many language-based tasks of school can be made accessible, and the classroom-based communicative needs of these children can be assisted.

4.1 Linguistic technologies for task assessment – reading tasks in particular

Before accommodating language needs, we of course need to assess students (bearing in mind all the assessment tools and assessment challenges discussed in Chapter 3). Besides the students themselves, we also need to assess the tasks they face. Gaps between task demands and existing skills then tell us where accommodations are needed.

As with remediation, so too with accommodation: the ultimate objective is to optimize learning. As discussed in the previous chapter, learning is optimized when tasks lie within students' zones of proximal development (ZPDs), the zones just between their current levels of mastery and what they can do only with help from others (see, for example, Engelmann 1999). The goal of task assessment and accommodation then is to ensure that the tasks faced by language-impaired students remain, to the greatest extent possible, within their respective ZPDs. In this, linguistic technology potentially plays several key roles.

One role is to help to identify the sometimes subtle linguistic demands of the various tasks that these students face, in particular, the many reading and writing tasks of school. Assessing a writing-based task automatically, via linguistic software, is far from straightforward. Somehow, the software would have to process the writing prompt (which is often rather open-ended) in ways that predict the linguistic demands of the associated task. Much more straightforward, or so it might seem, is the automatic assessment of reading tasks.

Reading difficulties, recall from Chapter 2, can occur in all the different developmental language disorders. Language comprehension deficits are generally independent of language modality: a child who struggles to understand words, sentences, and/or the implied meanings of particular uses of language will struggle whether those words, sentences, or uses occur in speech or in writing. Phonological deficits, meanwhile, impede the decoding of written words, and therefore, the entire reading process, limiting both frequency and fluency of reading. Furthermore, when decoding is not automatic, working memory is burdened. All these effects, in turn, can dampen comprehension and reading-based inferences.

Books and other texts are already assessed informally by teachers and formally by the standardized rating systems that label texts with grade levels. Recently joining these is the Lexile® Analyzer, a text-processing tool that assigns ratings to arbitrary texts. It measures two things: how challenging the individual words are (based on their frequency) and, as a proxy for syntactic complexity, how long the sentences are. The problem, however, is that sentence length correlates only weakly with the aspects of complexity that make sentence processing challenging (see, for example, Goodman & Freeman 1993; Just, Carpenter, Keller, Eddy & Thulborn 1996). A relatively long sentence may be quite easy to process if it consists of a series of simple short sentences conjoined with a coordinating conjunction like "and" ("I love you and you love me and we are a happy family"), while a relatively short "garden path" sentence like "The horse raced past the barn fell" can be quite difficult to process. Identifying the kinds of syntactic complexity that make reading challenging – particularly for children with specific language impairment (SLI) and autism – requires more sophisticated linguistic processing than that performed by the Lexile Analyzer.

An outline for how such a system might work, along with a crude version of it, is discussed in King and Just (1991). This system parses the sentences in a text and then uses the height of the parse tree (which indicates how much embedding there is), along with the number of clauses, noun phrases, and verb phrases per sentence, to provide an estimate of syntactic complexity. In principle, such a parser could be tweaked and normed for grade level, substantially improving upon the Lexile rating system. In particular, it might be tweaked to attend to different types of branching. Generally, right-branching sentences like "This is the cat that chased the rat that ate the cheese that lay in the house that Jack built", no matter how much embedding they contain, are easier to process than corresponding left-branching sentences like "The cat's prey's cheese's location's builder was Jack". Most challenging of all is what is called "center embedding", seen in sentences like "The cheese that the rat that the cat chased ate lay in Jack's house". Ideally, the parser should also attend to situations where there is initially more than one way to parse a sentence, as in "The horse raced past the barn fell".

There are, however, factors beyond vocabulary level and syntactic complexity that figure in text difficulty. These include the challenges of deducing the antecedents for the various pronouns and other anaphoric devices, including underspecified noun phrases like "that idea" and "this strategy". An automatic rating system might search for pronouns and deictics like "this" and "that" and compare the ratio of such terms to the number of noun phrases. A high ratio would indicate a highly interconnected, internally referential text that requires lots of inferences to determine antecedents and flesh out the content.

The amount of inferencing that readers must do, in fact, is a large part of how hard a text is. Beyond the inferences that determine antecedents for anaphors, there are a host of others, including the pragmatic inferences that make sense of dialogs, the social inferences that make sense of character interactions, and the perspective-taking inferences that make sense of actions in general. Such inferencing tasks are particularly challenging for children with autism. And yet, they pervade most reading assignments, especially fiction. They are the reason why reading fiction is one of the most demanding school-based tasks that children with autism face. But nonfiction is also challenging. Many texts, fiction and nonfiction, require yet another sort of inference: inferences that draw on general background knowledge. General background knowledge is the type of knowledge that most children pick up incidentally from social interactions and overheard conversations. Children with autism, less attuned to these sources of information, commonly have knowledge deficits, and therefore further deficits in reading comprehension.

To detect these inferencing demands, a linguistic software program would have to do precisely what eludes children with autism: identify any background knowledge assumed by the text and get inside the heads of any characters and look at the world of the text from their perspectives. But we are not even at a point yet where linguistic software can comprehend texts well enough to get inside their worlds, let alone the heads of the characters that exist there.

There are, nonetheless, cruder algorithms that might give rough estimates of social- and emotional-based inferencing demands. An automated text rater might search for social and emotional vocabulary terms and compute their density within the text. However imperfect a measure this is of the social- and emotional-based challenges for reading comprehension, it still would be a highly useful one, given that these challenges are a huge determiner of text difficulty for readers with autism and given that they do not figure at all in current text rating systems.

4.2 Linguistic technologies for classroom accommodation

Having played its role in assessing the linguistic skills of our language-impaired students and in rating the difficulty of tasks (particularly reading-based tasks), how might linguistic technology simplify tasks to match student' skills or otherwise make classrooms accessible?

Let us turn first to students with dyslexia. The task most impaired by this disorder, as discussed in Chapter 2, is reading. Most directly impaired is the decoding of written words into sounds. One obvious way to make reading tasks more accessible is to do the decoding for the student through text-to-speech (TTS) devices. Although most of these simply look up words in text-to-sound databases and use basic phonics rules to sound out unfamiliar words, more sophisticated linguistic processing devices, as discussed in Chapter 1, also use a text's punctuation to generate appropriate intonation. Combined with a speech recognition tool that automatically highlights the words in the text as they are read, such devices also potentially serve as teaching tools, helping dyslexic readers learn associations between printed words and sound. On the other hand, they potentially detract from time spent on activities that may be more beneficial in the long term, i.e. reading activities in which students practice letter-to-sound decoding on their own.

Speech-to-text devices, encoding text rather than decoding it, might also provide useful assistance to dyslexic students. In many cases, recall, difficulty decoding written words is accompanied by difficulty encoding words in writing. In spelling out words for students, speech-to-text devices might also, as with TTS devices, simultaneously serve as teaching tools and/or, conversely, reduce time spent on activities with greater long-term benefits (e.g. independent writing practice).

Returning to TTS devices, there is one more caveat to keep in mind. Some educators have assumed that these are helpful to all students who struggle with reading. As we have seen, however, the reading difficulties of children with SLI, autism, and other language delays have more to do with vocabulary, grammar, pragmatics, and inferences: converting a written text into speech will not alleviate these difficulties.

Indeed, in some cases, students with SLI and autism may do better with text than with spoken language – for example, if they have trouble orienting to speech, processing it fluently, or sustaining attention, as they often do. Speech, after all, is fleeting, while text-based transcriptions of speech allow repeated rereading. Some individuals with autism are more drawn to written symbols than to speech sounds, and some parents and teachers have observed that children with autism comprehend movies better when the subtitles are on. A speech-to-text device could potentially provide text transcripts of oral language in classroom settings – although the noisy environments and casual speech that predominate in classrooms would make this quite challenging. In combination with a directional microphone or FM system, the device could give a student a running transcript of what the teacher is saying, doing with the classroom what subtitles do with movies. Down the line, improved linguistic technology might enhance the quality of speech-to-text transcripts, allowing the processing not just of individual speech sounds, but also of intonation and syntax, using these linguistic cues to add appropriate punctuation, and thus additional clarity.

Turning now to deficits in vocabulary, while dictionary definitions are often only a mouse click away, a more carefully tailored device might provide in-context definitions. One of the challenges of dictionary definitions is the multiplicity of possible meanings. Word-sense disambiguation technology, deployed to process online texts, can select a word's most likely meaning in its given context. As with TTS technology in dyslexia, this feature might also foster word learning. It is important to remember, however, that definitions are limited in their ability to convey meaning. They show how words relate to other words (e.g. how "president" is a "leader" of a "country"), but not how they relate to the real world. As we noted earlier, if you do not already know what a "leader" and a "country" are, you still will not know what a "president" is.

As we have seen, the linguistic difficulties of many students with language impairments extend beyond vocabulary to phrases and sentences. In reading assignments, often it is the complexity of sentences that is most forbidding. So what about technologies that simplify sentences? With additional functionality, the software that Petersen (2007) proposes for analyzing a text's syntactic complexity might potentially simplify complex structures to make them more readable. This, of course, is something that teachers of language-impaired students can do, as the need arises, by hand. Simplified texts for classics like Shakespeare, furthermore, already exist. What automatic text simplification potentially offers, however, is speedy, on-the-spot simplification of arbitrary texts, including more recently published material, and specific passages within textbooks – even math textbooks – that may turn out to pose problems for particular students.

In actuality, text simplification software is only in its infancy, in some cases depending on manually simplified texts as training material (see Petersen 2007). The output of such programs, moreover, still requires manual editing. The two main strategies in text simplification are to remove adjectival and adverbial phrases and to remove subordinate clauses and convert them into separate sentences. Both methods have their downsides. Removing descriptive terms may remove details that either are important or make a text colorful and interesting. Converting clauses into separate sentences may simplify syntax but distort content. Consider "Sally thinks that the marble is in the basket". Taking "the marble is in the basket" out of its host sentence yields something like "Sally thinks something. The marble is in the basket". But what if the marble is actually in the box?

Furthermore, this kind of text simplification does not simplify inferences. Instead, it may multiply them. In stripping sentences of adverbs and adjectives and converting subordinate clauses into main clauses, text simplification may remove vital information that can be recovered only by inference. Syntactic simplification, in other words, may generally entail pragmatic complication. It may also increase demands on working memory. In general, the more compressed the information is, the more able we are to hang on to it. Consider "Sally thinks the marble is in the basket but Anne knows that it is in the box". Turned into four simple main clauses, the result is "Sally thinks something. The marble is in the basket. But Anne knows something. It is in the box". Aside from the additional inferencing required to deduce that "The marble is in the basket" is something that Sally thinks and that "It is in the box" is something that Anne knows, there is the additional strain of holding in working memory a longer stretch of discourse – four main clauses instead of two – and of deducing the antecedent of "it", which, now two sentences away, is much less obvious than before. For further discussion of the challenges of simplified language, see Goodman and Freeman (1993).

Automatic text simplification is even more elusory, as we discussed earlier in connection with text rating systems, when it comes to the myriad pragmatic and social inferences required for full comprehension. These, again, are what make reading most challenging to students with autism; addressing them is perhaps also the most challenging text simplification task of all.

4.3 Assistive communication technologies for developmental language disorders

Finally, what can technology do to assist students with their own communication, whether orally or in writing assignments?

Most in need of communicative assistance, of course, are children with the most severe language impairments: children who often have speech impairments in addition to productive language impairments. For this population, the most common assistive communication devices are those that use stored word and phrase recordings and/or TTS technology to convert user input into speech. User input usually occurs via arrays of word/icon buttons that are typically both pre-set to particular words, phrases, word categories, and situation categories (e.g. "cafeteria", "playground"), and customizable (by teachers, parents, and/ or the users themselves) to additional words, phrases, and categories that are important to particular users. The user selects from among these buttons, sometimes navigating through hierarchies of categories, and his selections are converted into pre-recorded or synthesized speech. The most common are the DynaVox Compass and Proloquo2Go. Figures 4.1 and 4.2 show two screenshots from the Proloquo2Go, and Fig. 4.3 shows a shot of the DynaVox Compass.

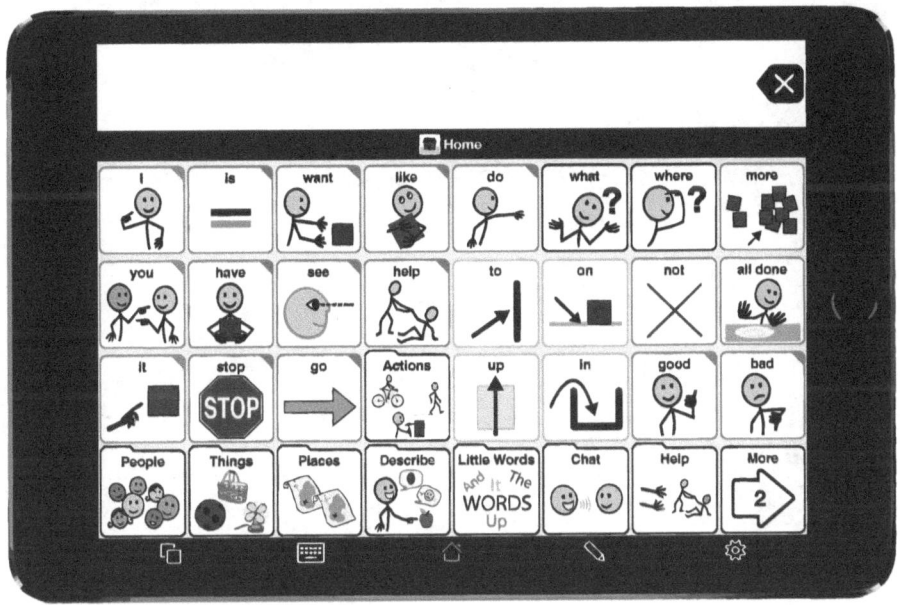

Fig. 4.1: Proloquo2Go home page.

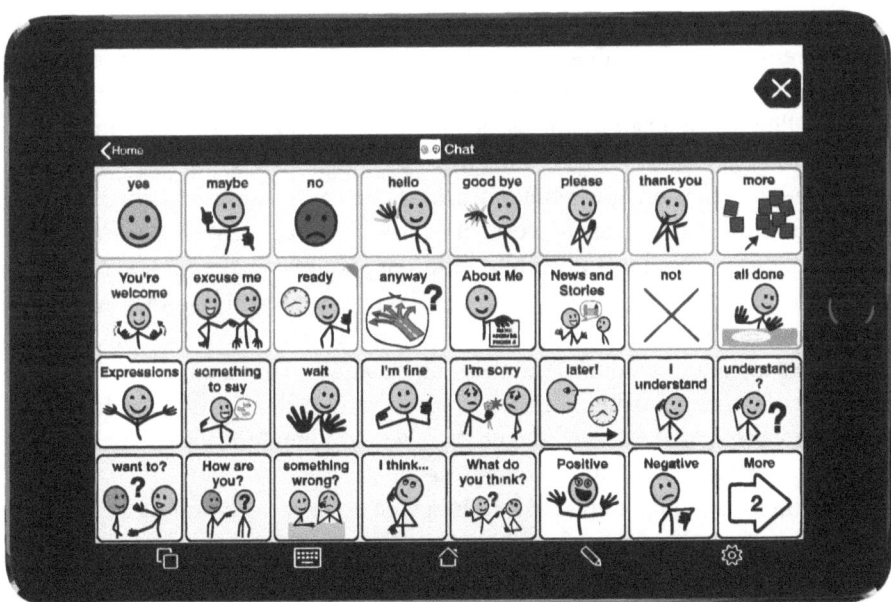

Fig. 4.2: Proloquo2Go chat page.

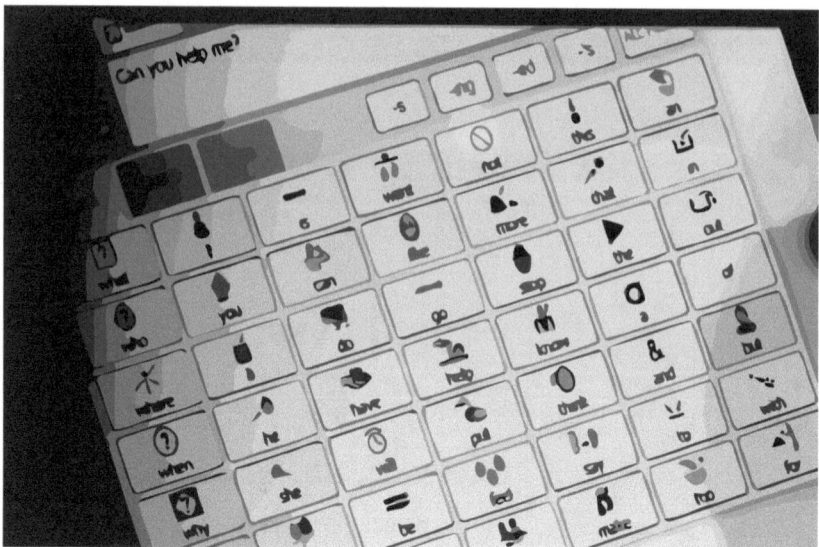

Fig. 4.3: DynaVox compass.

What these technologies do is enable children with speech and productive language impairments to bypass speech or vocabulary deficits and communicate basic requests, questions, and statements via icons: icons that are either quite transparent in their meanings or that the child (and his caregivers) have learned to associate with specific meanings or messages. In the course of using such devices, children may gradually associate the icons with their verbal labels, learning a number of sight words in the process.

Given the limits on how many word/icon choices these devices can display at a time, on how many levels of word categories are practicable for users to navigate through, and on how fully the situation categories cover the actual situations the child encounters in real life, these devices may not readily express everything a child might wish to communicate. On the other hand, the word hierarchies and categories are often customizable: they can be adjusted to maximize convenience for particular users. Furthermore, those who use these devices often lack the literacy and/or motor skills that would enable them to communicate via the infinitely more flexible medium of alphanumeric keyboards.

For those language-impaired children who do have keyboarding skills, there is a different type of assistive technology. Known as "text completion", "word prediction", or "word cue" software, it can be plugged into word processing programs on both laptops and tablets. It is also built into the DynaVox Compass and

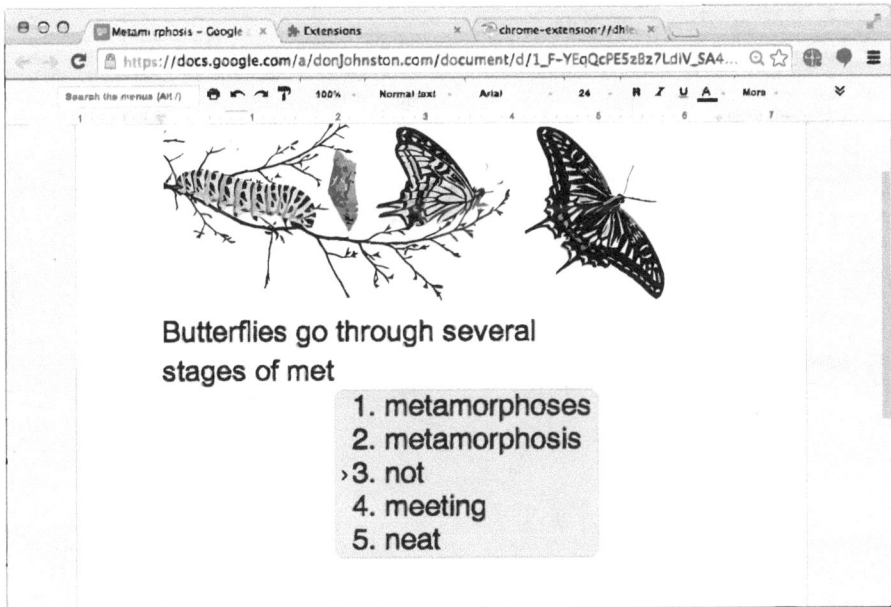

Fig. 4.4: Co:Writer word prediction.

Proloquo2Go – both of which offer keyboard interfaces in addition to word/icon buttons.

Text completion, in its most rudimentary form, is familiar to anyone who searches the Internet or uses an iPhone. Activated when the user begins typing, it guesses at the remaining letters of a word once enough of that word has been typed. More sophisticated programs start guessing earlier in the typing process, offering users lists of words to choose from. Figure 4.4 shows a screenshot of Co:Writer where just the first few letters instantiate choices.

An example from Penfriend, where the first letter has not even been typed, is shown in Fig. 4.5.

Figures 4.6 and 4.7 show two screenshots of Read&Write Gold, which offers an even longer list of choices.

The most popular programs (besides those built into Proloquo2Go and the DynaVox Compass) are WordQ, Aurora Suite, Classroom Suite, Soothsayer, Penfriend, Read&Write Gold, and Co:Writer – all of them usable with any standard writing software (e.g. Microsoft Word, WordPad, Notepad, or Outlook). The key ingredients of these programs are windows that pop up as the user types to propose likely next words. These proposals reflect what is

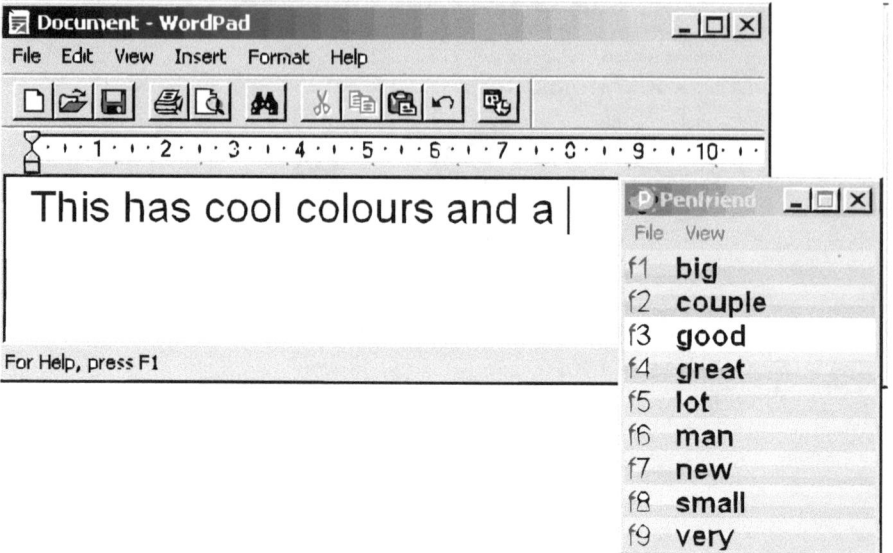

Fig. 4.5: Penfriend predictor.

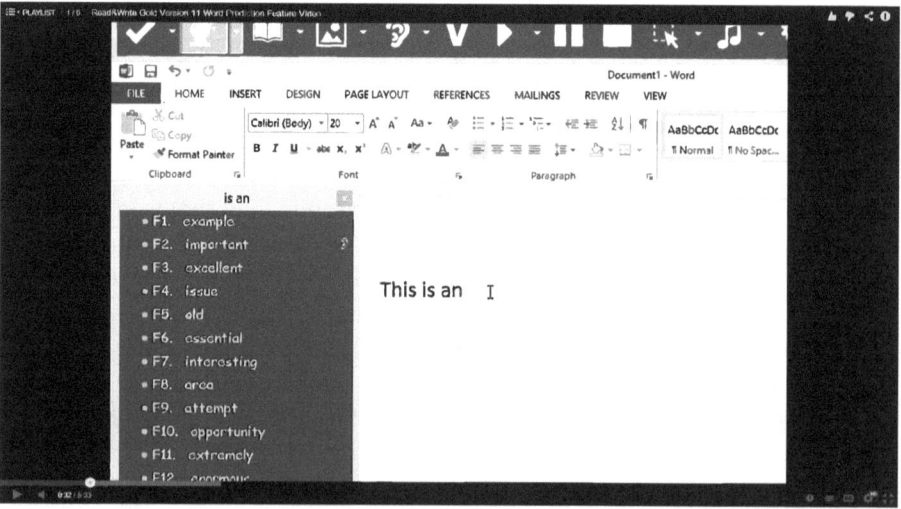

Fig. 4.6: Read&Write Gold word prediction.

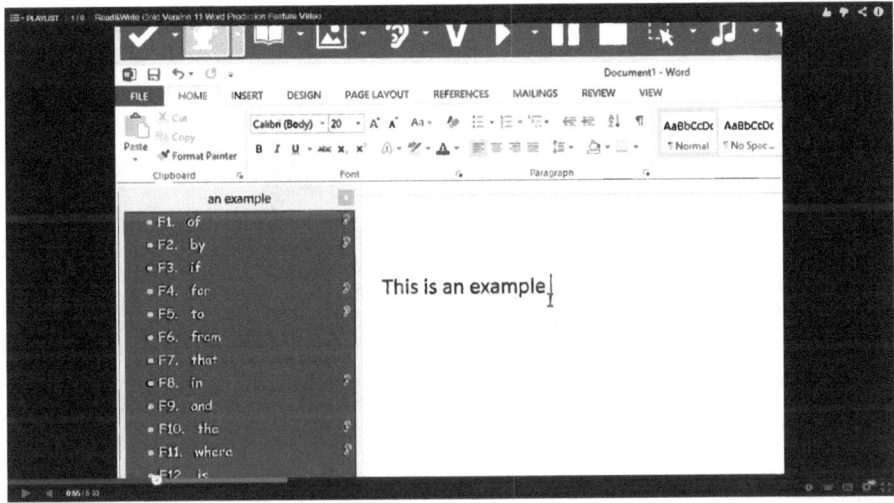

Fig. 4.7: Figure Read&Write Gold word prediction.

syntactically, morphologically, and/or semantically appropriate based on what the user has typed so far and on what is likely given general statistics about word occurrence, and in some cases (Read&Write Gold), the specific statistics that it collects on the word-selection habits of individual users. The software can read the selected words out loud; it can also echo back what the user has typed thus far, with highlighting, helping him or her detect typos and misspellings.

Some of these programs have additional features. In WordQ, a blanking out of the word list while one is typing flags typos or spelling mistakes. "Creative misspellings" (e.g. "rite") instantiate a pop-up list of alternative options. Co:Writer's FlexSpell feature guesses intended words from misspellings (Fig. 4.8).

The Read&Write Gold program has a dictionary that pops up when words from the list are highlighted, with examples of how the words might be used, and sometimes, visual illustrations. It also orders and highlights words according to likelihood and places a special icon next to words easily confused with other words. In addition, it allows users to select particular topics – topics as specialized as Polish architecture – and then calls up a topic-specific dictionary and topic-specific word choices (nouns, verbs, adjectives, etc.).

To help students who have no idea what to write about on a particular topic, Co:Writer displays a word bank, with words sized by topic relevance, as we see in Fig. 4.8.

To allow gradual fading of scaffolding, some programs (e.g. Co:Writer) permit administrators to turn off particular features – e.g. the grammatical predictions

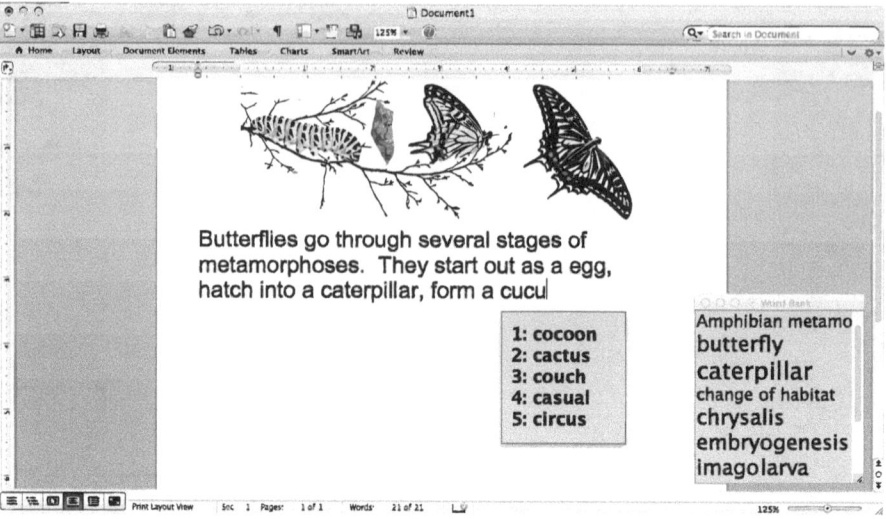

Fig. 4.8: Co:Writer Flexspell+word bank.

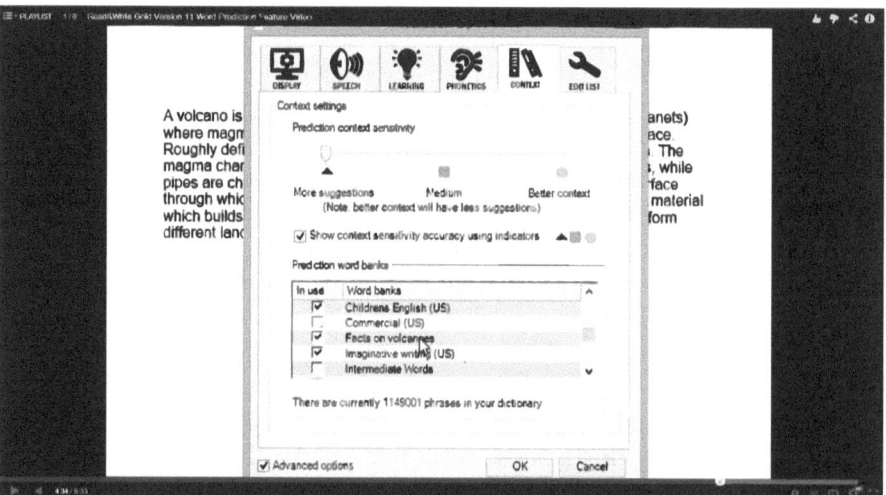

Fig. 4.9: Read&Write Gold settings.

within the text completion, and/or the automatic suggestions based on spelling errors, and/or the text-completion functionality in its entirety (Fig. 4.9).

Because it can read out loud the word choices as well as help with spelling errors, text-completion software is marketed specifically at students with dyslexia. But since spelling is a relatively minor part both of dyslexia and of text-completion software, this software potentially provides far greater assistance to children with other language deficits. In particular, it can help SLI students and grammar-impaired students with autism choose correct word forms and include grammatical function words. In some of the programs, for example, a student who types "I want" will see the word "to" as one of his or her choices, which steers him or her away from errors like "I want go". A student who types a plural subject like "my friends" will (depending on the program) only see verbs in the plural form (for example, "are" rather than "is"). A student who types "is" or "are" will (depending on the program) only see main verbs in the progressive or past participle form. A student who types the article "an" will (in some programs) only see noun choices that begin with vowels – as we see in Fig. 4.6. Or, as we see in Fig. 4.7, a student who types "an example" will (in some cases) see, as his or her first choice, the preposition that most often follows the word "example" ("of").

These programs thus offer significant help with spelling, with proper verb form, and with preposition agreement, as well as with coming up with what to say in the first place. Just like TTS and speech-to-text devices vis-à-vis dyslexia, text-completion devices also potentially serve as teaching tools, reinforcing correct syntax and word forms. On the other hand, they, like these other devices, potentially detract from activities that may be more educationally beneficial, like trying to figure out on one's own what the next word or word form should be, or what to write about on a particular topic.

Text-completion software still has room for additional linguistic sophistication. As we can see from some of the above images, for example, not all choices are grammatically correct or sufficiently informed by statistical frequency. Furthermore, the kind of natural language generation functionality discussed in Chapter 1 could increase the assistive power of text-completion in word/icon devices like Proloquo2Go and the DynaVox Compass – allowing it, for example, to suggest whole sentences rather than just next words. For example, when the user pushes the "cookie" button, the software could generate options like "I want a cookie" and "Do you want a cookie?", or if the user pushes the "he", "she", and "like" buttons, the system could offer options like "He likes her" and "She likes him". Such functionality potentially expands significantly the communicative flexibility of word/icon devices – and, possibly, the user's learning opportunities as well.

Another technology we all are familiar with, but which can serve in an assistive capacity, in particular, for children with grammar difficulties, are the autocorrections and the corrective feedback – squiggly, color-coded underscores – seen in programs like Microsoft Word. As this technology becomes more sophisticated, it, too, potentially provides significant grammatical help. It might, for example, automatically correct the main verb based on preceding auxiliaries, putting verbs that follow "is"/"are" in the progressive "-ing" form and verbs that follow "have" or "had" in past participle form. While squiggly lines, which prompt manual corrections, may also serve as teaching tools, autocorrections, which happen quickly and are easy to ignore, may be of more limited pedagogical value.

How efficacious are these software programs at their current level of sophistication? One thing to measure is their efficacy as teaching tools – for decoding and spelling words, or for using correct morphology and syntax. To what extent do they enhance learning, and to what extent do they detract from it? How helpful they are as assistive devices is perhaps harder to gauge. One option is to measure frequencies of usage and rates of abandonment, which is easiest to do in situations where users have to connect remotely to a designated server. Users might also be surveyed, although language impairments may limit responses. A third indicator of efficacy is teacher impression.

Outsider impressions as measures of efficacy raise an important caveat. When watching someone use text completion or word/icon-button software, it can be hard to tell how much she is capable of doing on her own vs. how much the software is doing for her. How much is she intentionally communicating rather than simply selecting – perhaps somewhat arbitrarily – among suggested words or icons? The checkered history of facilitated communication – in which it has turned out that it was mostly the facilitators, rather than the students, who were doing the communicating – should keep parents, therapists, and educators vigilant about where the child leaves off and the assistive device takes over. Even if the child, alone, is responsible for the communicative content of the facilitated messages, how much of the morphology and syntax is his own? Unless one takes the time to assess their unassisted communication skills, one may assume that students are doing more than they are actually capable of doing. We will revisit this concern in Chapter 5, where we propose various caveats about developmental language technology.

References

Engelmann, S. (1999). Student-program alignment and teaching to mastery. In *25th National Direct Instruction Conference*.

Goodman, K. & Freeman, D. (1993). What's simple in simplified language? In: Tickoo M, ed. *Simplification: Theory and application* (pp. 69–76). Singapore: SEAMEO Regional Language Center.

Just, M. A., Carpenter, P. A., Keller, T. A., Eddy, W. F. & Thulborn, K. R. (1996). Brain activation modulated by sentence comprehension. *Science, 274*, 114–116.

King, J. & Just, M. A. (1991). Individual differences in syntactic processing: The role of working memory. *Journal of Memory and Language, 30*, 580–602.

Petersen, S. E. (2007). *Natural language processing tools for reading level assessment and text simplification for bilingual education*. Doctoral dissertation, University of Washington, Seattle, WA.

Katharine Beals

5 Conclusions and caveats about developmental language technology

Abstract: This chapter concludes the portion of the book that is devoted to developmental language disorders. It reviews what to look for, and what to look out for, in selecting linguistic technologies for particular developmental language disorders, and for particular remediation or accommodation goals.

We have reached an exciting point in the development of linguistic technology for developmental language disorders. Never before have speech therapists, teachers, parents, and children themselves had so many tools to choose from. But the large number of technologies, and the variation in services they provide, quality they exhibit, and costs they impose (ranging from a few dollars to many hundreds of dollars), mean that determining which technology to provide to which child involves a fair amount of reflection and research. Given that using linguistic software also involves an often large time commitment on the part of the student and his or her family, making an uninformed choice can waste not just money but also time: time that could be spent using better software and reaping better results. This is where a knowledgeable speech therapist can play an invaluable role: helping parents and teachers make good choices about software.

What do good choices involve? When it comes to remediation software in particular, it is important to ensure that the skills taught are the ones the particular child actually needs help with. Children with certain forms of SLI need disproportionate help with comprehension; those with other forms of SLI need disproportionate help with syntax. Children with autism often need both; some only need help with pragmatics. Children with dyslexia need help primarily with phonemic awareness and word decoding.

After you have determined what skills a particular child needs to develop, the next step is to compare these skills both with the stated goals of particular software programs and with what skills they address in practice. Does the program, on close inspection, really teach what it says it does? Beware especially of lavish claims and customer testimonials: often, the skills taught are considerably narrower than what is suggested on websites and in other promotional materials. Some programs that claim to teach grammar, for example, have not been reviewed here in this book as grammar teaching programs because, in fact, they only teach vocabulary and specific phrases. Other programs that purport to teach certain sentence structures, as we have seen, only teach comprehension (and sometimes only partial comprehension) of these structures, not the details of how to produce them.

Then there is the issue of efficacy. As it turns out, most programs lack convincing data. Some companies cite efficacy studies, but these often turn out to be unpublished monographs about studies conducted by individuals affiliated with the company in question. Or, even if the studies have been published, their authors include company affiliates and their results have not been replicated by independent researchers. Often, the number of experimental subjects is quite low – i.e. in the single digits. Methodological flaws are common. For linguistic software in particular, efficacy testing must take into account that children, in the course of normal development and everyday exposure to language, not to mention any additional language therapies that they may be undergoing, often experience linguistic progress independently of training. A comparison of linguistic improvements in areas specific to training with improvements in other aspects of language, using one or more of the standard language assessments discussed in Chapter 3, is crucial to tease out which effects are training-specific. For example, if the software trains children in sentence structure rather than in vocabulary, standardized language tests administered after training would be expected, assuming the training was effective, to show relatively greater progress on syntax subtests than on vocabulary subtests.

Finally, even when studies are well-designed, are well-controlled, and do show convincing efficacy results, these results are often confined to progress within the software program itself. The real questions are whether the skills taught will be retained, and more importantly, whether they will generalize to real-world situations. As a meta-analysis of autism software in general (not just language software) has shown, precisely this sort of generalization is frequently lacking (Wass & Porayska-Pomsta 2014).

This does not mean that no linguistic software programs are effective. To some extent, the dearth of efficacy studies simply reflects the myriad obstacles to conducting well-designed, publishable studies. Language learning is a long process; linguistic software interventions often take many weeks, or months, to administer; proper administration and supervision take many man-hours. Recruiting and retaining reasonable numbers of subjects, including control subjects, is challenging; so, too, is locating training venues and finding funding sources for administration and supervision. Researchers who are unaffiliated with the software company may have little incentive to conduct studies. The upshot: we should not assume that an absence of convincing efficacy studies means an absence of actual efficacy.

In the absence of convincing efficacy studies, how else might one determine which programs show promise? One can look for online reviews on sites other than the company's own website, especially on sites that contain honest, critical, comparative reviews of a variety of related products. One can look for opportunities to see the software in action without purchasing it. Often companies provide demos of their programs; one can try these out with potential candidates. If the company does not provide demos online or on request, or at least provide videos showing the program in use (one place to look for these is YouTube), it is reasonable to question whether the program is as promising as claimed.

Other red flags are specific to certain types of programs. With programs that claim to teach grammar, there are several things to watch out for. Is the main focus really on grammar and its general rules and structures, or is it on vocabulary and specific phrases? If the program does focus on general rules, are these the kinds of grammar rules that language-impaired students need help with and that have been our focus throughout this book – word order and word endings – or are they the kinds of rules aimed at all students – part of speech labels, rules specific to the standard dialect, and the conventions of written language (punctuation, the spelling of homophones, and rules of style). Here, it is important to distinguish between "school grammar", also called "prescriptive grammar", which many students need help with, and the more basic grammar discussed throughout this book, which only language-impaired students need help with.

Once you have ensured that the latter sort of grammar is addressed by the program, there are additional questions to ask. Does the program teach this grammar explicitly, or merely provide incidental exposure? Incidental exposure may still be effective, but, as discussed in Chapter 3, it is impossible to ensure that the user is paying attention. Does the program teach productive grammar or only receptive grammar? Receptive grammar is worth instructing in its own right, but, as discussed in Chapter 3, mastery of particular receptive grammar skills does not guarantee mastery of corresponding productive grammar skills. Finally, if the program teaches productive grammar, how wide a range of structures does it teach and how much of the grammatical work is done for the student instead of by him?

Programs that purport to teach pragmatics should also raise red flags. As we have seen, the vast majority of pragmatics, open-ended and dependent on real-life contexts as it is, is ill-suited to computerized learning. A program like Simmersion, for all its virtual reality features, does not present users with practice making the kinds of open-ended choices in novel situations that real life requires. Relatedly, some people consider pragmatics to be primarily about figurative language, and figurative language, in turn, to be characterized by phrases like "It's raining cats and dogs" and "Can you pass the salt?" But the meanings of these phrases, while not literal, are still readily predictable: "raining cats and dogs" always means "raining heavily"; "can you pass the salt?" nearly always means "pass the salt". A program that teaches the meanings of such phrases is therefore more like a vocabulary program than a pragmatics program. Aside from set expressions like these, and the regular rule-based pragmatics of deictics and pronouns (see Chapter 3 for discussion), face-to-face, in-person therapy may be the best modality for explicit pragmatics instruction.

Let us turn now to accommodation. Whether or not we are looking at linguistic technologies in particular or at accommodation strategies in general, it is important to beware of the potential pitfalls of either over- or under-accommodating. Ideally, we want tasks to fall within a child's zone of proximal development – the zone just between her current level of mastery and what she can do only with help from others. It is hard to get this right, but crucial to try.

Under-accommodation may result from a faulty first step: a faulty assessment of task demands. Especially for children with autism, tasks may present subtle challenges that fly under the radar of neurotypical people, teachers included. Perhaps most commonly overlooked in language-based tasks (for example, reading assignments) are subtasks that require the socio-emotional inferences or use of general background knowledge (see Chapter 4 for discussion) that come naturally to individuals without autism. It is important to remember that rating scales, including automatic rating scales like the Lexile® Analyzer, do not take these challenges into account. A book that looks quite easy to others, and that rates low on the Lexile scale, may still be quite challenging to students with autism.

Then there is the possibility of over-accommodating and not sufficiently challenging the child. Text-completion software in particular raises this possibility, potentially putting words in the child's mouth that she is capable formulating independently.

As far as text completion and other assistive communication technologies go, the inherent uncertainty on the part of outside observers about how much students are doing on their own vs. how much the software is doing for them is yet another concern. To what extent are users intentionally communicating rather than simply selecting – perhaps somewhat arbitrarily – among suggested words or icons? Might we be overestimating their communicative skills? Might there be more to remediate than we realize?

And how does this affect everyone's incentives – particularly the incentives of students and teachers? In general, the more efficacious the assistive technology appears to be, the more it potentially reduces the urgency of teaching and practicing the skills that are being assisted. Text-to-speech (TTS) devices potentially reduce the incentive to teach decoding skills for reading; they may also reduce the incentive for students to work on their reading skills by actually reading. Speech-to-text devices, similarly, may reduce the incentive to teach and practice spelling skills. Assistive communication devices and text-completion software in turn may reduce the incentive to teach and practice independent communication skills. It is essential that assistive technology be treated only as such – namely, as assistive – and not as grounds for reducing remediative instruction and practice.

A final concern pertains to children with autism in particular: the extent to which technology takes these children, already diminished in their social interactions, away from the face-to-face exchanges on which they may be especially dependent for their social and socio-pragmatic development. Screens, as we have observed, are no substitute for the pragmatics of open-ended, real-world interactions. But too often, whether or not the students are autistic, one finds classrooms and other settings in which students are mostly looking at and interacting with screens rather than with one another.

Heightening these concerns are two things. One is the proliferation of technology in the classroom, with purchasing decisions made by individuals or committees who are often insufficiently informed about educational value and efficacy, especially where special needs students are concerned. The other is the unprecedented pressure that today's schools and teachers are experiencing. In the United States, most language-impaired students are included in regular classes with same-aged peers, and these classrooms are under increasing pressure to teach to the new Common Core State Standards and tests. In English and Language Arts, these standards set high expectations for reading and writing and take a one-size-fits-all approach to students at a given, typically age-based, grade level (see Beals 2014). In light of this, fewer and fewer teachers, even special education teachers, feel that they have time to remediate basic skills – especially when the growing prevalence of assistive devices makes remediation seem ever less urgent. Indeed, some of the assistive technology websites, e.g. Classroom Suite, explicitly mention the Common Core standards as motivating their use in the classroom (see Intellitools).

In fact, remediation and accommodation should go hand in hand. The ultimate goal, after all, is to optimize the learning environment such that students reach their potential, and, ultimately, are liberated from assistive technology to the largest extent possible.

We conclude this chapter with a recap of key caveats:
1. Keep up to date on the many emerging new technologies via frequent and thorough web searches.
2. Do a thorough assessment of each child's linguistic weaknesses. Different language impairments require different interventions and remediations.
3. Compare the goals that you want to achieve with the stated goals of the software and with what it actually seems to teach.
4. Beware of lavish claims of skills taught, particularly where grammar and pragmatics are concerned.
5. Beware of claims of efficacy. Look for published, peer-reviewed, well-designed studies, especially by authors who are unaffiliated with the software company.

6. Check whether the efficacy results include generalization to real-world situations.
7. Do not assume that a lack of efficacy studies means that a particular program is ineffective.
8. Especially if efficacy studies are lacking, request and try out software demos.
9. Beware of the limitations of automated text rating systems in rating texts for difficulty.
10. Remember that many reading difficulties stem from comprehension problems rather than decoding problems and cannot be alleviated with TTS devices.
11. Beware of the pitfalls of under- and over-accommodation.
12. Beware of the fine line between remediation and accommodation. Make sure that technologies like TTS, speech-to-text, and text completion do not reduce commitment to the teaching and learning of independent skills.

References

Beals, K. (2014). The common core is tough on kids with special needs. *The Atlantic Online*.

Intellitools. Retrieved from http://www.ablenetinc.com/Assistive-Technology/IntelliTools/Classroom-Suite

Wass, S. V. & Porayska-Pomsta, K. (2014). The uses of cognitive training technologies in the treatment of autism spectrum disorders. *Autism: International Journal of Research and Practice, 18*, 851–871.

Ruth Fink

6 Overview of acquired aphasia and disorders of word retrieval

Abstract: Chapter 6 begins our discussion of aphasia and aims to provide the reader with a general understanding of the impairments and psychosocial consequences associated with this devastating communication disorder that results from stroke or other injury to the brain. Because aphasia can affect all language processes (speaking, reading, writing and understanding speech) to varying degrees, it has a profound affect on a person's ability to fully participate in everyday life activities. Noting that word retrieval deficits are the hallmark of aphasia, the author explains the different types of word retrieval deficits and provides an overview of treatment approaches.

6.1 Aphasia

"Aphasia" is an acquired language impairment caused by stroke or other neurological disorder. Aphasia can affect language expression (spoken and written) and language comprehension (spoken and written). Aphasia symptoms vary considerably across patients and have been described in numerous ways. One approach is to classify aphasia syndromes into two broad categories: fluent aphasia and non-fluent aphasia. Within each category individuals are further distinguished by their performance on measures such as auditory comprehension, repetition, and verbal production. Assessment of verbal production includes naming ability (including type of naming error), grammatical performance, articulatory agility, and prosody (Goodglass & Kaplan 1983).

6.1.1 Fluent aphasia

Individuals with fluent aphasia typically produce sentence-like utterances with normal or near-normal intonation and articulatory agility. However, each of the four types of fluent aphasia (Wernicke's aphasia, transcortical sensory aphasia, conduction aphasia, and anomic aphasia) has unique patterns of strength and weakness in the domains of comprehension and verbal expression.

Wernicke's aphasia, for example, is characterized by deficits in auditory-phonological processing. The result is poor auditory comprehension with fluent, sentence-like utterances that resemble English rhythm and syntax but contain "words" or "nonsense words" filled with phonological errors, rendering much of the speech jargon-like (think Lewis Carroll's *Jabberwocky*). Speech is often rapidly produced and picture naming responses contain phonological errors, word substitutions and omissions. Self-monitoring is typically poor. Reading and writing are also impaired, but perhaps to a lesser extent. Grammatical errors (paragrammatism) in spoken and written production are also present.

In contrast, individuals with anomic aphasia have good auditory comprehension, and fluent, grammatical speech but notable difficulty in word finding. While there may be some phonological errors and word substitutions during production, most errors are frequent use of empty, nonspecific words (e.g. "thing", "this here"), descriptions of the intended word ("it is for your head" for "hat"), or failure to retrieve a word. "I know it but I can't say it" is a frequent response. Repetition of single words is usually good, and many individuals with anomia may be able to recognize errors, but not able to correct them ("it is a bed, no") much of the time.

6.1.2 Non-fluent aphasia

Individuals with non-fluent aphasia (Broca's aphasia, transcortical motor aphasia, global aphasia) exhibit limited speech output. Broca's aphasia, for example, is characterized by halting speech, with impaired prosody and articulatory agility. Verbal production consists of short, agrammatic utterances composed primarily of nouns and other content words. Auditory comprehension is superior to verbal expression, and while comprehension of single words and conversation is good, comprehension of syntactically complex sentences is typically impaired. Noun naming is often superior to verb naming. Non-fluent agrammatic aphasia will be discussed in depth in chapter 9. A complete description of aphasia diagnostic categories can be found in *Common Classifications of Aphasia*.

6.1.3 Living with aphasia

Although aphasia affects a person's ability to speak, read, write, and comprehend speech to varying degrees, it does not affect intelligence. People with aphasia know more than they can say or communicate. Aphasia also does not affect memory in the way that dementing conditions do. However, the everyday consequences of aphasia are profound. For those with severe aphasia, simply communicating basic needs is a challenge. Impairments in speaking, reading, and writing make everyday tasks (e.g. speaking or reading to their children, helping with homework, following printed recipes, sending and reading messages via e-mail, Facebook, or other social media) difficult, if not impossible. Therefore, most individuals with aphasia are unable to return to their former occupations or fully resume household and family responsibilities. Many lose touch with family and friends, causing further isolation. Although some people with aphasia have substantial spontaneous recovery over a period of weeks or months, many will experience a persistent aphasia that is likely to be a lifelong chronic disability.

According to the National Aphasia Association (www.aphasia.org), one in three stroke survivors will have aphasia. It is estimated that more than 2 million people in the United States live with aphasia, and there are more than 200,000 new cases each year in the United States alone.

6.2 Disorders of word retrieval in aphasia: "I know it but I cannot say it"

While aphasia symptoms vary depending on the location and extend of the brain damage, word retrieval deficits are the most common impairment in aphasia and are found in all of the syndromes described above. Word retrieval deficits also manifest in different ways, and most researchers and clinicians broadly differentiate between word retrieval deficits that are primarily semantic (meaning based) or phonological (sound-based) in nature. A meaning-based error (e.g. saying "table" for "chair") is also referred to as a semantic paraphasia. A sound-based error (e.g. saying "sencil" for "pencil") is also called a literal or phonemic paraphasia. When numerous sound errors are present in a word, it is termed a neologism or jargon.

Psycholinguistic models of word production provide a useful framework for understanding the nature of the impairment and differentiate several subtypes, including (1) semantic deficits, characterized by semantic errors in word comprehension and verbal production (e.g, saying "table" for "chair"); (2) phonological retrieval deficits, in which access to phonology from semantics is impaired and thus characterized by good comprehension, word substitutions, descriptive responses (saying "it is that thing that you write with" when shown a picture of a pen) or absent responses in picture naming ("it is a ... " or "I know it but I can't say it"); and (3) phonological encoding deficits, characterized by good comprehension, with phonological errors in naming, repetition, and/or oral reading. However, as with all aphasic syndromes, these subtypes are rarely pure and patients often exhibit a combination of deficits. For example, individuals with primarily phonological encoding problems might not only produce a greater proportion of phonological errors, but also exhibit semantic errors in naming. Others may not only exhibit good lexical comprehension for single words but show comprehension deficits when tested with more sensitive measures. (For a recent review of research on models of word retrieval and the semantic-phonological interaction in lexical access, see Schwartz 2014).

The following speech samples illustrate the varying characteristics of a naming disorder in three individuals with different types of "fluent aphasia" who are describing a picnic scene from the Western Aphasia Battery (Kertesz 1982).

Sample 1: Person without aphasia

> In this picture it looks like a family is enjoying the day, outside by a lake, A man and woman are sitting on a blanket, under a tree and having a picnic lunch. The man is reading a book while the woman is pouring a drink. A picnic basket and radio are on the blanket. Another person, maybe a friend, is flying a kite, and a dog is playing next to him. Someone is fishing from the dock, someone is sailing a boat and someone is wading in the water.

Sample 2: Person with anomic aphasia (S1)

> Ok. There are ... a man and a woman. Sitting in a ... sitting outside and having a picnic ... and he's playing a book, he's reading a book ... and she's /r-/ and she's drinking some ... something to drink. And ... they're sitting outside ... in this in this area that has a bunch of ... grass and ... stuff outside and there's a man outside and he's /f-/ doing a kite. And ... he's he's got his kite out there, he's playing his kite. And there's a dog sitting next to him. And there's ... a little boy that's outside. He's down toward the end ... of ... the the grassy area. Just sitting down there probably playing. Because there's um ... there's uh ... (I don't know what this is called) ... (I don't know) and then there's some people up here ... in um ... they're in uh ... I don't know what that is either. I don't know, sorry.

In the above sample, we see that S1 speaks in well-articulated, grammatical sentences, but has frequent difficulty retrieving content words (e.g. nouns, verbs, adjectives). In her attempts to describe the picture, there are frequent pauses (...) while she searches for words, self-corrections, substitutions of words, omissions of words, false starts, descriptions, and failure to retrieve, resulting in absent or general responses. S1 knows what she wants to say, but is unable to retrieve the words in a timely manner. She is aware of her errors, but not always able to consistently self-correct. S1 has good comprehension of speech (input semantics), will recognize the correct word when she hears it and reject incorrect words, and is able to repeat words, but has difficulty with finding the words to express her thoughts.

The presumed breakdown in her word retrieval system is in accessing the phonological word form from semantics (a so-called phonological retrieval problem).

Sample 3: Person with Wernicke's aphasia (S2)

> well someone he here this right … they are in their (kas) there to uh a one, (shurnecks) one with a (wini) and one with a (nekster) over here, someone sitting foot (bunz) by the run, he's got a knife, someone uh what is that? … I can't /?/ do but she's doin' with the rest and a right uh the right things, it's very (wenel) you know, just one out there and the (ti), um this guy is (red) off and his glasses, this oh someone's (tiken) it's (timen) over there, uh she's in a (ormernef) for is (dif) it's like a little thing for that, um that kind of thing?

S2 is a person with a Wernicke's aphasia. As can be seen, utterances are fluent and sentence-like but devoid of informative content words and filled with empty speech, verbal and phonemic paraphasias, and neologisms (words in parentheses are neologisms). His picture description is produced with appropriate intonation and articulation. He is unable to repeat words correctly, demonstrates poor single-word auditory comprehension, and has difficulty following conversation. Self-monitoring is poor. Written word comprehension and production is better, but still impaired, and his written output (not shown here) is paragrammatic, with numerous grammatical errors.

Sample 4: Person with conduction aphasia

> This boy is … is usin' it's um … a /gaɪt/ (galt) a /gaɪt/ (galt) uh I can't get the name of it. Uh a /kaɪk/) kite … fan is /run-/ I mean a /f-/ fan … fun … .(fag) (fein). The boy in there is sittin' in here … and puttin' fishes in that I mean … the fishing right here … the boy is in here watchin' um … the /b-/ um … a /b-/ a bucket in um … the sand. This is a right here is um … a /b-/ a /b-/ a /s-/ a boat … a boat … a whatever call it in there (rawl). Um. Tryin' … uh man I can't get the words out.

As can be seen in the above sample, this person often has a word in mind, but makes multiple phonological errors as he struggles to get the intended word out (the so-called conduit d'approche). Comprehension is good as is self-monitoring. Unlike the person with anomic aphasia who is able to repeat words, this person is unable to use repetition to aid production. In fact, impaired repetition is a typical marker of this subtype of aphasia.

In summary, all people with aphasia have some type of word-finding difficulty, although failure to retrieve a word will result in different error patterns, depending on whether the deficit is more or less semantically or phonologically based.

6.3 Approaches to treating word production disorders in aphasia

Not surprisingly, much treatment research has studied differences between semantic approaches, which focus on strengthening semantic processing of words, and phonological approaches, which aim to improve access to the word form and phonological production. A review of the literature reveals that both approaches have been shown to be beneficial and that in many studies the protocols invoke both semantic and phonological processing (for a review and discussion, see Nickels & Best 1996a,b; Nickels 2002; Raymer & Rothi 2002), although the emphasis may be more or less on one or the other. Most speech language pathologists use a combination of approaches to treat the broad range of symptoms that they see in the clinical setting. Below we describe some examples of each type of treatment that has been studied and shown to have beneficial effects.

6.3.1 Lexical-semantic treatments

Lexical-semantic treatments typically aim to strengthen access to semantic features and word meanings. Semantic tasks, which have been used in treatments and shown to be effective, include spoken or written word-picture matching tasks, categorization tasks, semantic feature selection, making relatedness judgments, and synonym selection. For examples of these treatments, see Howard, Patterson, Franklin, Orchard-Lisle and Morton (1985a,b), Marshall, White-Thompson and Pring (1990), Boyle and Coelho (1995), Nickels and Best (1996a,b), Coelho, McHugh and Boyle (2000), Boyle (2001, 2004), and Kiran and Bassetto (2008), and for a review, see Nickels (2002) and Kiran and Bassetto (2008).

  We illustrate one popular treatment called Semantic Feature Analysis (SFA). SFA and its variants have been the subject of a number of studies (e.g. Boyle & Coelho 1995; Coelho et al. 2000; Boyle 2001, 2004). Treatment involves the presentation of a picture and subsequent questions to generate feature information about the targeted picture. The picture is placed in the center of a page and spaces are provided to fill in information about the word's features as each is elicited, including its group (what category is it), use (it is used for ...) properties (visual description), location (where you find it), association (it reminds me of ...). Once all of the features have been elicited either verbally or by multiple-choice selection, participants are asked to name the picture. If still unable to name the picture, the participant is asked to repeat the name after the examiner.

SFA is hypothesized to work by strengthening connections between a word and its semantic network, thus raising the threshold for activation and subsequent naming. Findings from a number of studies show that this training typically improves naming of treated and untreated words and gains are typically maintained.

6.3.2 Lexical-phonological treatments

Phonological treatments aim to facilitate the retrieval and production of the phonological word form using tasks that facilitate production and attention to the word's phonological and/or orthographic form. Phonological tasks that have been beneficial include phonological (and orthographic) cueing of picture names, word repetition, analysis of a word's phonological components (e.g. rhyme, first sound, final sound, number of syllables), and oral reading. For examples of these treatments, see Micelli, Amitrato, Capasso and Caramazza (1966), Raymer, Thompson, Jacobs and Le Grand (1993), Hillis and Caramazza (1994), Robson, Marshall, Pring and Chiat (1998), Hickin, Herbert, Best, Howard and Osborne (2002), Martin, Fink, Laine and Ayala (2004), and Leonard, Rochon and Laird (2008).

In one phonological approach, Leonard et al. (2008) developed a phonologically based treatment that was modeled after SFA. Following the protocol of Coelho et al. (2000), a target picture is placed in the center of a chart and participants are asked to identify a series of phonological components for that target: a rhyme, the first sound, final sound, number of syllables. Participants may select a response from a list if unable to generate the response independently. Treatment effects were positive for 7 of the 10 participants, gains were maintained at 4 weeks post-treatment, and some generalization was reported to untreated items. In a follow-up study, van Hees, Angwin, McMahon and Copeland (2013) compared SFA and PCA in eight people with aphasia and found that the phonological protocol resulted in beneficial effects for seven of eight participants, while the semantic protocol resulted in positive effects for four of eight participants. Interestingly, the semantic protocol was not beneficial for patients with semantic deficits, while the phonological protocol was beneficial for participants with both deficits.

6.3.3 Semantic and phonological tasks are rarely pure

It has been pointed out that semantic and phonological treatments are rarely pure (Howard 2000; Nickels 2002). In the "phonological" task described above, for example, the picture is usually present, thus providing semantic information. In semantic tasks such as word-picture matching or SFA treatment, the spoken or written form of the word is typically provided and the patient may be asked to name or repeat the name of the picture. Raymer and Rothi (2002) and Nickels (2002) concluded that the most effective naming treatments should encourage both semantic and phonological processing within the same treatment protocol, since that is in keeping with current models of word production where there are multiple levels of processing that engage when a word is selected and produced. In the clinical setting, it is common practice to test a variety of cues (semantic, phonological, orthographic, and gestural) to determine which cue is facilitative for a given person. Often, a hierarchy of cues is provided, as seen in the studies of Linebaugh and Lehner (1977) and Thompson, Raymer and Le Grand (1990).

In the next chapter, we briefly review selected treatment studies that have implemented some of these techniques on the computer.

References

Boyle, M. (2001). Semantic feature analysis: The evidence for treating lexical impairments in aphasia. *Neurophysiology and Neurogenic Speech and Language Disorders, 112*, 23–28.

Boyle, M. (2004). Semantic feature analysis treatment for anomia in two fluent aphasia syndromes. *American Journal of Speech-Language Pathology, 13*, 236–249.

Boyle, M. & Coelho, C. A. (1995). Application of semantic feature analysis as a treatment for aphasic dysnomia. *American Journal of Speech-Language Pathology, 4*, 94–98.

Coelho, C. A., McHugh, R. E. & Boyle, M. (2000). Case study: Semantic feature analysis as a treatment for aphasic dysnomia: A replication. *Aphasiology, 14*, 133–142.

Common classifications of aphasia. Retrieved April 3, 2015, from http://www.asha.org/ Practice-Portal/Clinical-Topics/Aphasia/Common-Classifications-of-Aphasia/

Goodglass, H. & Kaplan, E. (1983). *The Assessment of Aphasia and Related Disorders (2nd Edition)*. Philadelphia, PA: Lea & Febiger.

Hickin, J., Herbert, R., Best, W., Howard, D. & Osborne, F. (2002). *Efficacy of treatment: Effects on word retrieval and conversation*. Hove, UK: Psychology Press.

Hillis, A. & Caramazza, A. (1994). *Theories of lexical processing and rehabilitation of lexical deficits*. Hove, UK: Lawrence Erlbaum.

Howard, D. (2000). Cognitive neuropsychology and Aphasia therapy. The case of word retrieval. In I. Papathanasiou (Ed.), *Acquired neurogenic communication disorders: A clinical perspective*. London: Whurr.

Howard, D., Patterson, K., Franklin, S., Orchard-Lisle, V. & Morton, J. (1985a). The facilitation of picture naming in aphasia. *Cognitive Neuropsychology, 2*, 49–80.

Howard, D., Patterson, K., Franklin, S., Orchard-Lisle, V. & Morton, J. (1985b). Treatment of word retrieval deficits in aphasia: A comparison of 2 therapy methods. *Brain, 108*, 817–829.

Kertesz, A. (1982). *Western Aphasia Battery*. San Antonio, TX: The Psychological Corporation.

Kiran, S. & Bassetto, G. (2008). Evaluating the effectiveness of semantic-based treatment for naming deficits in aphasia: What works? *Seminars in Speech-Language Pathology, 29*, 71–82.

Leonard, C., Rochon, E. & Laird, L. (2008). Treating naming impairments in aphasia: Findings from a phonological components analysis treatment. *Aphasiology, 22*, 923–947.

Linebaugh, C. & Lehner, L. (1977). *Cueing hierarchies and word retrieval: A treatment program.* Minneapolis, MN: BRK Publishers.

Marshall, J. P. C., White-Thompson, M. & Pring, T. (1990). The use of picture/word matching tasks to assist word retreival in aphasic patients. *Aphasiology, 4*, 167–184.

Martin, N., Fink, R., Laine, M. & Ayala, J. (2004). Immediate and short-term effects of contextual priming on word retrieval. *Aphasiology, 18*, 867–898.

Micelli, G., Amitrato, A., Capasso, R. & Caramazza, A. (1966). The treatment of anomia resulting from output lexical damage: Analysis of two cases. *Brain and Language, 52*, 150–174.

Nickels, L. (2002). Therapy for naming disorders: Revisiting, revising, and reviewing. *Aphasiology, 16*, 935–980.

Nickels, L. & Best, W. (1996a). Therapy for naming disorders (Part 1): Principles, puzzles and progress. *Aphasiology, 10*, 21–47.

Nickels, L. & Best, W. (1996b). Therapy for naming disorders (part II): Specifics, surprises and suggestions. *Aphasiology, 10*, 109–136.

Raymer, A. M. & Rothi, L. J. G. (2002). Clinical diagnosis and treatment of naming disorders. In A. Hillis (Ed.), *The handbook of adult language disorders: Integrating cognitive neurospsychology, neurology and rehabilitation* (pp. 163–182). Philadelphia: Psychology Press.

Raymer, A. M., Thompson, C. K., Jacobs, B. & Le Grand, H. R. (1993). Phonological treatment of naming deficits in aphasia: Model based generalization analysis. *Aphasiology, 7*, 27–53.

Robson, J., Marshall, J., Pring, T. & Chiat, S. (1998). Phonological naming therapy in jargon aphasia: Positive but paradoxical effects. *Journal of the International Neuropsychological Society, 4*, 675–686.

Schwartz, M. F. (2014). Theoretical analysis of word production deficits in adult aphasia. *Philosophical Transactions of the Royal Society B, 369*, 20120390.

Thompson, C. K., Raymer, A. M. & Le Grand, H. R. (1990, June). Effects of phonologically based treatment on aphasic naming deficits: A model-driven approach. In *Clinical Aphasiology Conference*, Santa Fe, NM, USA.

van Hees, S., Angwin, A., McMahon, K. & Copeland, D. (2013). A comparison of semantic feature analysis and phonological components analysis for the treatment of naming impairments in aphasia. *Neuropsychologic Rehabilitation, 23*, 102–132.

Ruth Fink

7 Software for aphasia: computer-assisted treatment of word retrieval deficits in aphasia

Abstract: In chapter 7 the author continues a discussion of treatment for aphasia and introduces research software and commercial products that are designed to enhance and intensify treatment for aphasia. The author provides a brief survey of the evidence for computer-assisted treatment of word retrieval deficits.

7.1 Technology for aphasia: what are the benefits?

Computer technology, if used to its potential, offers enormous payoffs for this population. Although there is no cure for aphasia, research has shown that, under the right circumstances, progress can continue for many years following the initial injury and that language therapy is beneficial even many years post onset (e.g. Fink, Brecher, Schwartz & Robey 2002; Salter, Teasell, Foley & Allen 2013). The importance of treatment intensity has been established in a number of studies (for a review, see Bhogal, Teasell & Speechley 2003; Basso 2005), yet clinical practice rarely allows for intensive or long-term treatment, largely due to restrictions in insurance reimbursement. Now that advances in technology make it possible to implement many effective treatment protocols on the computer, there is greater opportunity to extend the rehabilitation process, increase the intensity of practice, and improve the efficiency of therapy – all considered important for gains to continue. Additionally, barriers to communication can be reduced with the use of assistive technology such as text-to-speech, word prediction programs, and picture-based communication software. Many programs are now available as apps for use on smartphones and/or tablet and costs are more affordable. However, to promote maximum use and benefit, we need computer software with user-friendly interfaces, evidence-based protocols, and automatic feedback. This is crucial to dealing with the long-term needs of our clients.

7.2 Language software for aphasia: what is the evidence?

Computers are now widely used in aphasia therapy, and there is a growing body of experimental literature that attests to the benefits of these various programs [for example, Lingraphica, a multidomain program (Aftonomos, Steele & Wertz 1997); Oral Reading for Language in Aphasia (ORLA) (Cherney 2010); Aphasia Scripts™ (Cherney, Halper, Holland & Cole 2008); MossTalk Words® for word retrieval deficits (Fink, Brecher, Schwartz and Robey, 2002); Sentactics®, for sentence production deficits (Thompson, Choy, Holland and Cole, 2010); SentenceShaper® (SentenceShaper 2015), for sentence production (Linebarger, Schwartz & Kohn 2001); for reading (Katz & Wertz 1997); Constant Therapy 2015, a multidomain program (Kiran, Des Roches, Balachandran & Ascenso 2014); Aphasiamate™, a multidomain program (Archibald, Orange & Jamieson 2009)]. However, large clinical trials demonstrating their efficacy are sparse. Many popular commercial programs (e.g. Parrot Software 2015, Bungalow, Morespeech, TalkPath, and Tactus TherAppy) have exercises based on tasks typically used in therapy and report anecdotes of success and satisfaction, but have themselves not undergone experimental evaluation of their efficacy, (but see Corwin, Wells, Koul and Dembowski (2014), who demonstrated improvement in naming and oral discourse following the use of specific Parrot software programs). In the past 5 years, there has been an explosion in the development of apps and web-based programs for aphasia. A recent special issue of *Seminars in Speech and Language* (Kurland 2014) is devoted to the issues and promises of using tablet-based technology in rehabilitation of aphasia. A current list of aphasia software and apps can be found at http://aphasiasoftwarefinder.org, an aphasia-friendly website.

In the area of word retrieval, a number of researchers have implemented computer-based programs that replicate what has been successful in therapy and have demonstrated positive outcomes (for a review, see Van de Sandt-Koenderman 2004; Fink, Brecher, Sobel & Schwartz 2005; Van de Sandt-Koenderman 2011). Below, we summarize some of the studies and illustrate the types of tasks that have been studied.

Providing the first sound of a word (phoneme cueing), for example, often facilitates word production for many people with phonological retrieval deficits. Additionally, some people with aphasia are able to provide the first letter of a word they are unable to say. Based on this knowledge, Bruce and Howard (1987) developed a computer-generated treatment that converted letters to sounds to provide self-generated cues. Following treatment, all participants demonstrated improvement in naming treated and untreated items when the aid was used. In a subsequent study, Best, Howard, Bruce, and Gatehouse (1997) used the same computer-generated cueing procedure with another, more severe patient, who had limited letter knowledge and found significant and long-term improvement for treated and untreated items even without use of the aid.

Multicue, developed by Van Mourick and Van de Standt-Koenderman (1992), offers patients a variety of cueing options (phonological and semantic), with a goal of enabling patients to integrate successful word-finding strategies to access words. Of the first four patients treated with Multicue, one made significant gains in naming test scores, two made modest gain and one patient made no gains. In a follow-up study by Doesborgh et al. (2004), 18 individuals were randomized to Multicue (n = 8) or no treatment (n = 11). Only the treatment group showed improvement in naming test scores as measured by the Boston Naming Test (Goodglass, Kaplan & Weintraub 1983).

Adrian, Gonzales, and Buiza (2003) report on the effectiveness of the Computer-assisted Anomia Rehabilitation Program in a single case study. Sixty words were targeted for treatment over 12 sessions. Different types of cueing were used systematically across the treatment sessions (phonological, semantic, written, and mixed). Results showed significant gains on treated and non-treated items that were maintained on testing at 1 month post-treatment.

Some computer-assisted treatments focused on written naming and found improvement in both written and oral naming. Deloche, Dordain, and Kremins (1993) studied two patients with different underlying impairments. The therapist selected the cues (semantic or phonological) based on the participant's impairment profile. Pictures and cues were presented simultaneously and the patient responded by typing the correct name. If incorrect on two successive attempts, the computer automatically provided feedback in written form. There was no oral training or auditory feedback. Both patients improved in written items and showed varying generalization patterns. For patient 1, improvement generalized to untreated items in both written and spoken modalities; for patient 2, generalization was noted for untrained items in written modality and trained items in oral modality.

Pedersen, Vintner, and Olson (2001) also demonstrated the effectiveness of written naming practice to improve oral naming. Additionally, this computerized treatment program was administered to three individuals without supervision, although each individual was provided with a computer pre-programmed with a set of tasks selected for each individual. Treatment focused on written naming. The programs included semantic tasks (e.g. spoken and printed word-picture matching with semantic foils), phonological tasks (e.g. printed word-picture matching tasks with phonological foils), and written tasks (e.g. copying, arranging anagrams, and writing unassisted). All patients showed varying degrees of improvement on written production of trained words as well as in oral naming. The patient with a primary phonological deficit showed the greatest gains, suggesting to the authors that phonological deficits could improve using a written approach.

Evidence that patients can benefit from independent or minimally supervised computer use come from several studies, including Laganaro, Di Petro, and Schnider (2003), who studied independent use in both chronic and acute patients; Mortley, Wade, and Enderby (2004), who used the Internet to deliver computer therapy for word retrieval deficits and monitored users remotely (see also Wade & Mortley 2003, and more recently, Palmer et al. 2012).

Additional evidence that computer-assisted treatment is beneficial and that independent work on the computer can be effective comes from a number of studies that involved a computerized therapy system called MossTalkWords®, which was specifically designed to be used in the clinical setting as well as by patients working independently.

In the following section, we provide an in depth look at the program, review the evidence for this program and then discuss a new version that integrated speech recognition into the program.

References

Adrian, J., Gonzales, M. & Buiza, J. (2003). The use of computer-assisted therapy in anomia rehabilitation: A single-case report. *Aphasiology, 17*, 981–1002.

Aftonomos, L. B., Steele, R. & Wertz, R. (1997). Promoting recovery in chronic aphasia with an interactive technology. *Archives of Physical Medicine and Rehabilitation, 78*, 841–846.

Archibald, L., Orange, J. B. & Jamieson, D. (2009). Implementation of computer-based language therapy in aphasia. *Ther Adv Neurol Disord, 2*, 299–311.

Basso, A. (2005). How intensive/prolonged should an intensive/prolonged treatment be? *Aphasiology, 19*, 975–984.

Best, W., Howard, D., Bruce, C. & Gatehouse, C. (1997). Cueing the words: A single case study of treatments of anomia. *Neuropsychological Rehabilitation, 7*, 105–141.

Bhogal, S. K., Teasell, R. & Speechley, M. (2003). Intensity of aphasia therapy, impact on recovery. *Stroke, 34*, 987–993.

Bruce, C. & Howard, D. (1987). Computer-generated phonemic cues: an effective aid for naming in aphasia. *British Journal of Language and Communication Disorders, 22* (3), 191–201.

Bungalow. www.bungalowsoftware.com

Cherney, L. (2010). Oral Reading for Language in Aphasia (ORLA): Evaluating the efficacy of computer-delivered therapy in chronic nonfluent aphasia. *Topics in Stroke Rehabilitation, 17*, 423–431.

Cherney, L. R., Halper, A. S., Holland, A. L. & Cole, R. (2008). Computerized script training for aphasia: Preliminary results. *American Journal of Speech-Language Pathology, 17*, 19–34.

Constant Therapy. (2015). www.constanttherapy.com

Corwin, M., Wells, M., Koul, R. & Dembowski, J. (2014). Computer-assisted anomia treatment for persons with chronic aphasia: Generalization to untrained words. Journal of Medical Speech-Language *Pathology, 21*, 149–163.

Deloche, G., Dordain, M. & Kremins, H. (1993). Rehabilitation of confrontation naming in aphasia: Relations between oral and written modalities. *Aphasiology, 7*, 201–216.

Doesborgh, S., Van de Sandt-Koenderman, M., Dippel, D., van Harskamp, F., Koudstaal, P. & Visch-Brink, E. (2004). Cues on request: The efficacy of multicue. A computer program for wordfinding therapy. *Aphasiology, 18*, 213–222.

Fink, R. B., Brecher, A., Schwartz, M. F. & Robey, R. R. (2002). A computer implemented protocol for treatment of naming disorders: Evaluation of clinician-guided and partially self-guided instruction. *Aphasiology, 16*, 1061–1086.

Fink, R. B., Brecher, A., Sobel, P. & Schwartz, M. F. (2005). Computer-assisted treatment of word retrieval deficits in aphasia. *Aphasiology, 19*, 943–954.

Goodglass, H., Kaplan, E. & Weintaub, S. (1983). The Boston Naming Test. Philadelphia: Lea & Febiger.

Katz, R. C. & Wertz, T. (1997). The efficacy of computer-provided reading treatment for chronic aphasic adults. *Journal of Speech, Language, and Hearing Research, 40*, 493–507.

Kiran, S., Des Roches, C. A., Balachandran, L. & Ascenso, E. (2014). *Seminars in Speech and Language, 35*, 38–50.

Kurland, J. (ed.) (2014). Tablet-based technology in the rehabilitation of aphasia. *Seminars in Speech and Language Pathology, 35* (1).

Laganaro, M., Di Pietro, M. & Schnider, A. (2003). Computerised treatment of anomia in chronic and acute aphasia: An exploratory study. *Aphasiology, 17*, 709–721.

Linebarger, M. C., Schwartz, M. F. & Kohn, S. E. (2001). Computer-based training of language production: An exploratory study. *Neuropsychological Rehabilitation, 11*, 57–96.

Morespeech. www.morespeech.com

Mortley, J., Wade, J. & Enderby, P. (2004). Superhighway to promoting a client-therapist partnership? Using the Internet to deliver word-retrieval computer therapy, monitored remotely with minimal speech and language therapy input. *Aphasiology, 18*, 193–211.

Palmer, R., Enderby, P., Cooper, C., Palmer, R., Enderby, P., Cooper, C., Latimer, N., Julious, S., Paterson, G., Dimairo, M., Dixon, S., Mortley, J., Hilton, R., Delaney, A. & Hughes, H. (2012). Computer therapy compared with usual care for people with long-standing aphasia poststroke: A pilot randomized controlled trial. *Stroke, 43*, 1904–1911.

Parrot Software. (2015). http://www.parrotsoftware.com

Pedersen, P. M., Vintner, K. & Olson, T. S. (2001). Improvement of oral naming by unsupervised computerised rehabilitation. *Aphasiology, 15*, 151–169.

Salter, K., Teasell, R., Foley, N. & Allen, L. (2013). Aphasia. In *Evidence-based review of stroke rehabilitation* (16th edition). http://www.ebrsr.com/evidence-review/14-aphasia

SentenceShaper®. (2015). http://www.sentenceshaper.com

Tactus TherAppy. www.tactustherapy.com

Talkpath. www.aphasia.com/talkpath

Thompson, C., Choy, J., Holland, A. & Cole, R. (2010). Sentactics®: Computer-automated treatment of underlying forms. *Aphasiology, 24* (10), 1242–1266.

Van de Sandt-Koenderman, M. (2004). High-tech AAC and aphasia: Widening horizons. *Aphasiology, 18*, 245–263.

Van de Sandt-Koenderman, M. (2011). Aphasia rehabilitation and the role of computer technology: Can we keep up with modern times. *International Journal of Speech Language Pathology, 13*, 21–27.

Van Mourick, M. & Van de Sandt-Koenderman, M. (1992). Multicue. *Aphasiology, 6*, 179–183.

Wade, J. & Mortley, J. (2003). Talk about IT: Views of people with aphasia and their partners on receiving remotely monitored computer-based word finding therapy. *Aphasiology, 17*, 1031–1056.

Ruth Fink and Deborah Dahl

8 Software for aphasia: MossTalk Words® (MTW)

Abstract: Chapter 8 continues the discussion on software for aphasia with an in-depth description and discussion of MossTalk Words, a computer-assisted treatment that incorporates a speech recognition feature. The authors share their experience as software developers of this research product and then expand the discussion to other software and apps that use speech technologies to aid and support everyday communication, including text to speech and speech to text technologies. The chapter provides a glimpse of how speech technologies are used in research, clinical and real life settings to reduce barriers and improve communication for people with aphasia.

8.1 About MossTalk Words: a computer-implemented treatment

MossTalk Words® (MTW), developed by Fink, Brecher, Montgomery and Schwartz (2001), provides extensive practice in word comprehension and production using multimodality cues and feedback. MossTalk's two main treatment modules, *Cued Naming* (CN) and *Multimodality Matching* (MMM) were modeled after treatments that are typically used by clinicians and have been shown to be effective in non-computerized experimental studies (e.g. word-picture matching (Howard, Patterson, Franklin, Orchard-Lisle & Morton 1985a, b); hierarchical cueing (Linebaugh & Lehner 1977; Thompson, Raymer & Le Grand 1991)). As such, they are designed to address both semantic and phonological deficits.

The program was designed to assist speech and language pathologists in efficiently selecting and delivering therapy exercises and tracking results. It was also designed for independent home use by language-impaired individuals and provides hours of practice in comprehending and producing words, phrases, and sentences. The system uses a large, easily customized vocabulary of words and pictures that is presented in multimodalities (auditory, visual). Exercises can be developed and accessed through several interfaces, each designed for a particular user.

The interface shown in Fig. 8.1 begins the selection process. The **standard** interface allows clinicians to quickly select the module (core vocabulary, CN, or MMM) and the particular exercise they wish to work on. When users select a vocabulary category (e.g. animals, objects, actions, mixed category), the program automatically presents a random set of words from the selected category. The **custom** interface allows the clinician (or family member) to pre-select

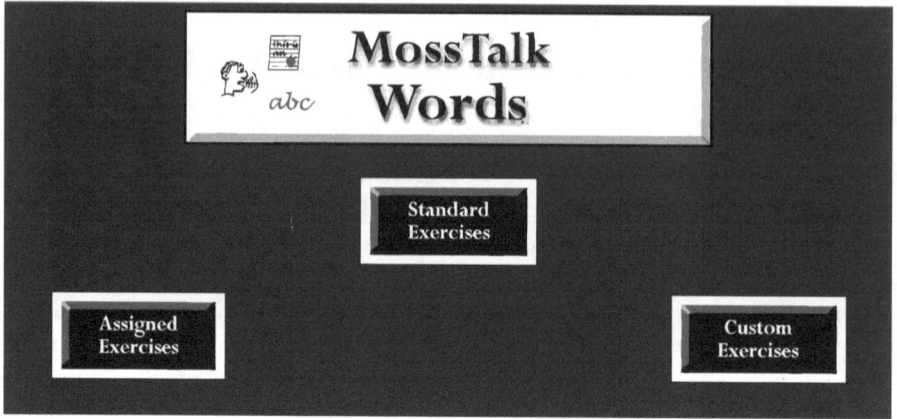

Fig. 8.1: MossTalk Words Select exercise interface.

specific vocabulary items from any category, thus affording users greater control over the vocabulary to be practiced in a given exercise. The **assigned exercises** interface enables clinicians (or others) to pre-select a set of exercises for patients to access independently later. Each module can be customized along a number of parameters (nouns or verbs, word frequency, semantic category, modality of presentation, number of stimuli on the screen). Performance is automatically tabulated and saved. A summary of the results can be displayed and/or printed.

The standard interface consists of three therapy modules (described below). Within each module, multiple exercises are organized in a hierarchy of difficulty, from easier to harder. Easier exercises employ high-frequency vocabulary, or in the case of multiple-choice exercises, fewer and/or less confusable choices (e.g. semantically unrelated foils); harder exercises present lower-frequency vocabulary and greater and/or more semantically related choices.

1. Core vocabulary module – a series of matching and naming exercises for the more severely impaired patient, involving a restricted vocabulary of words with high functional significance (e.g. names of foods, clothing, everyday objects).
2. Multiple choice matching module – a series of spoken and written word-picture matching exercises to facilitate comprehension and vocabulary development using pictures, spoken, and/or printed words, as shown in Fig. 8.2.
3. CN module – a series of exercises to facilitate single word production using a hierarchy of spoken and written cues.

Throughout the exercises, there is much opportunity for multimodality cueing and feedback. The CN module, (see Fig. 8.3), has four verbal cue options (first phoneme, sentence completion, definition, and spoken word). The same cues

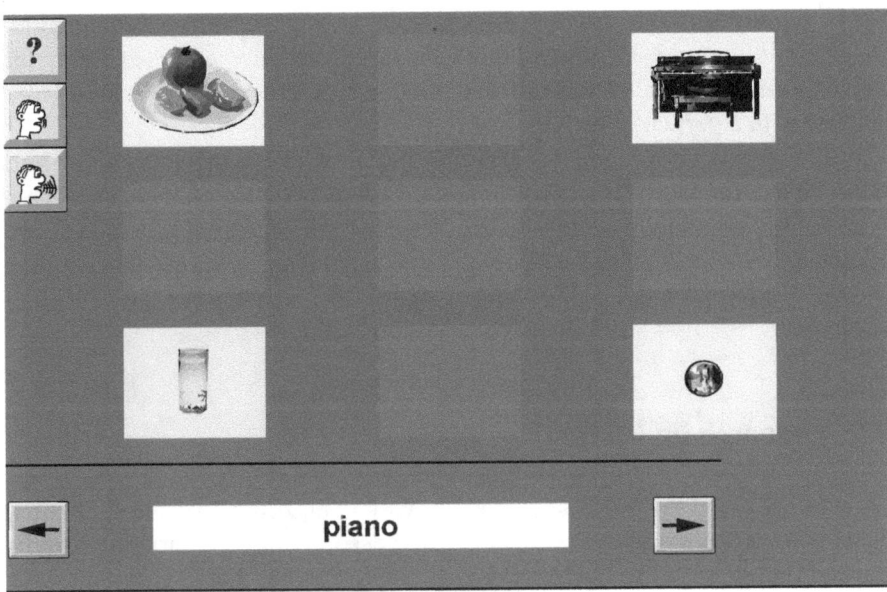

Fig. 8.2: MossTalk Words Written word-picture matching module.

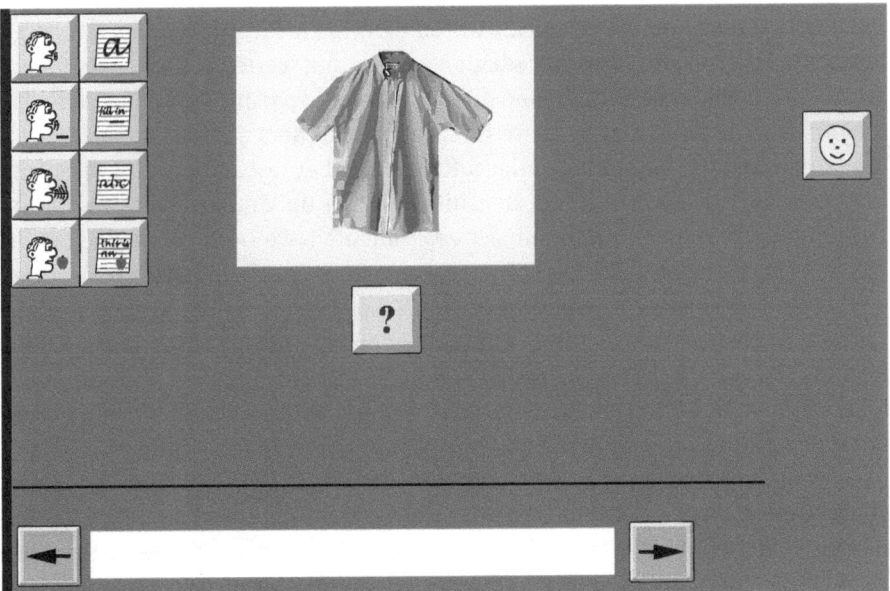

Fig. 8.3: MossTalk Words Cued Naming module.

can be presented in the print mode (i.e. first letter, written sentence completion, etc.). In addition to selecting the difficulty level, modality, and vocabulary for a given exercise, the clinician can also select which cues to activate for a given exercise with a particular patient.

In the original CN module (Fink et al. 2001), users are shown a picture and asked to say the word that corresponds to the picture. If unable to retrieve a word, users were taught to click on one or more of the eight spoken and written cues to help them recall the word. When a correct response was produced, they clicked the happy face to hear "that's right". Responses were automatically tabulated.

8.2 Research on MTW

An initial study of MossTalk's CN module (Fink et al. 2002) involved six participants with moderate-severe phonologically based naming impairment. Results showed that it was effective in improving naming skills, that participants were able to use the program with minimal guidance, and that independent work on the computer could be an effective adjunct to clinician-guided therapy. Clinical experience and use and satisfaction data collected from clinicians and patients (Sobel, Fink & Schwartz 2000) lent support to the experimental findings and provided evidence on the practicality of integrating MTW into a clinical therapy program. Importantly, the data demonstrated that patients and their family members – even those with limited prior computer exposure – could learn to use the program. Encouraged by these findings, researchers at Moss Rehabilitation Research Institute disseminated the software to other researchers and clinicians for further independent study. As a result, MTW has undergone extensive testing. Together, more than 17 single-subject experiments have been conducted on clinically relevant aspects of the software, including: its effectiveness for various etiologies and language symptoms (Raymer, Kohen & Saffel 2006; Jokel, Cupit, Rochon & Leonard 2006; Jokel, Cupit, Rochon & Graham 2007; Jokel, Cupit, Rochon & Leonard 2009; Raymer, Carwile, Matthews, Johnson & Todd 2009; Jokel, Rochon & Anderson 2010), its effectiveness when self-administered (Fink et al. 2002; Ramsberger & Marie 2005, 2007), and the impact of therapy intensity on outcomes (Ramsberger & Marie 2005; Raymer et al. 2006). In summary, these studies found that (1) both the CN and MMM modules improved naming (acquisition and maintenance) of trained words; (2) the software was effective with varied populations, including non-fluent progressive aphasia, semantic dementia, and moderate-severe chronic aphasia – both semantic and phonologically based; (3)

participants benefited when treatment was self-administered; (4) there was some benefit for greater intensity, but the benefits were variable across participants.

8.3 Speech recognition in MTW-2

In the original version of MTW, whether the user correctly named the object presented or not was assessed by either a clinician or the user. Although that method of assessing correctness was usable, it was thought that incorporating a speech recognition feature into the software would further enhance its therapeutic flexibility and user acceptance and make it a more powerful clinical and research tool, since it could then automatically record responses and provide feedback in the absence of a research assistant or clinician. Accordingly, speech recognition capability was added to MTW. Instead of self-assessing whether the picture was correctly named or not, speech recognition software would compare the user's speech to the expected word and decide if the spoken response was correct. Since MTW was already running in a Windows environment, we selected the speech recognizer built into Windows (Windows Speech Recognition) as our recognition technology. We faced several usability challenges in the design of the speech recognition feature.

Users' speech might be distorted from normal speech in ways that would make the recognizer fail, even if the user correctly named the picture. If the clinical goal is to encourage the user to improve their pronunciation, this would be desirable, but if the clinical goal is to simply assess whether the user had correctly named the picture, it would be better if the recognizer was more forgiving about the user's pronunciation. To accommodate varying clinical goals, the user interface to MTW includes a slider to control the recognizer confidence and a checkbox for whether or not common phonological errors should be accepted. With those settings, the clinician, user, or family member can adjust the strictness of the recognizer. A screenshot of this interface is shown in Fig. 1.12 of Chapter 1.

1. Even a correctly pronounced word might not be recognized, which could be frustrating for the user. To address this we used several strategies.
    a. A special, aphasia-friendly training process was developed so that the recognizer could adapt to the user's speech because the normal Windows Speech Recognition training process is too difficult for most aphasic users.
    b. The recognizer was controlled by a grammar that was only expecting the target word, minor phonological variations of the target word, and synonyms of the target word, greatly constraining the recognizer's task, thereby improving its accuracy.

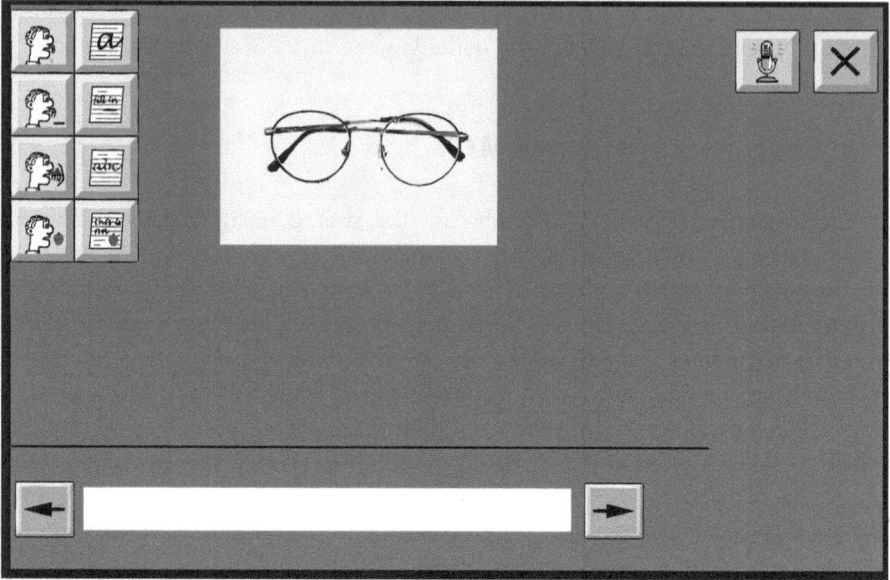

Fig. 8.4: MossTalk Words user interface with speech recognition.

    c.   An "objection" button was developed so that the user could note a recognition error in the record keeping.

    d.   The recognition feature was made optional, so that users could proceed without using it if they found it frustrating.

Figure 8.4 shows the MTW user interface with speech recognition enabled. The smiley face for self-assessing the user's performance on naming has been removed, since the recognizer will be doing the assessment in this version of MTW. Two user interface features have been added. The microphone button turns the microphone on or off (it is important to be able to turn off the microphone to prevent unintended audio from triggering the speech recognizer) and the objection button (the X) has been added to allow the user to record disagreement with the recognizer. A white circle (not shown) indicates that the recognizer has heard some sound. If the sound was not recognized as the target word, nothing else happens, and the system simply waits for the user to speak again or to proceed to the next picture. However, if the correct word was recognized, the system will play a tone and then say, "That's right!"

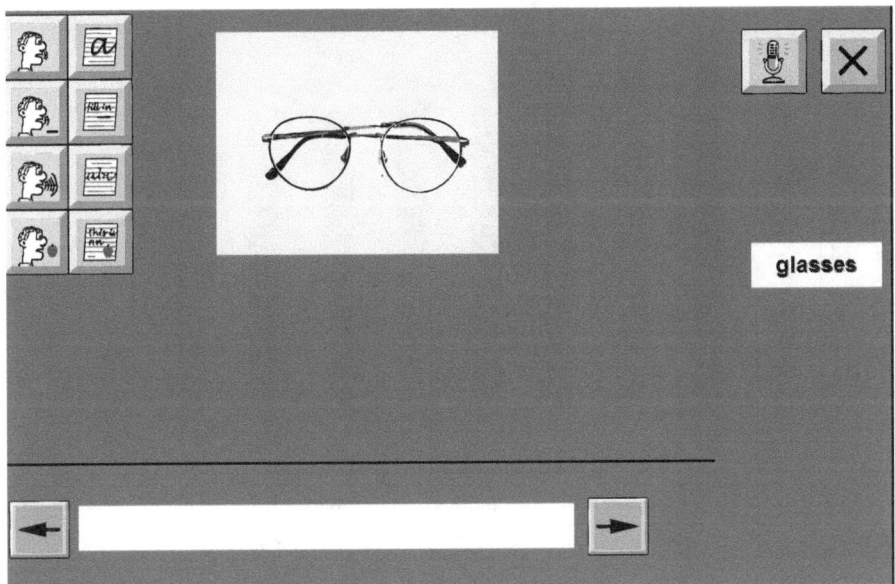

Fig. 8.5: MossTalk Words user interface after successful speech recognition.

along with the name of the picture. It will also present the written name of the picture for additional reinforcement. The user interface after a successful recognition is shown in Fig. 8.5.

We evaluated MTW-2 with several studies testing users with aphasia (Fink, Schwartz & Dahl 2009; Fink & Dahl 2012). While the full details of the studies are out of the scope of this book, we generally found that the recognition worked reasonably well for most users and that users had a high level of satisfaction (on a five-point scale) with the speech recognition feature, even for the users who were not recognized very well (e.g. S3, S4) as shown in Fig. 8.6.

We also found that recognition accuracy improved when the participants began training the recognizer with the user's individual profile. For S3, the recognizer's percent accuracy rate for correct responses following four training sessions increased to 0.96. At follow-up testing, recognition accuracy remained at 0.96. For S4, the recognizer's percent accuracy rate following four training sessions increased to 0.86. At follow-up testing, recognition accuracy was 0.94.

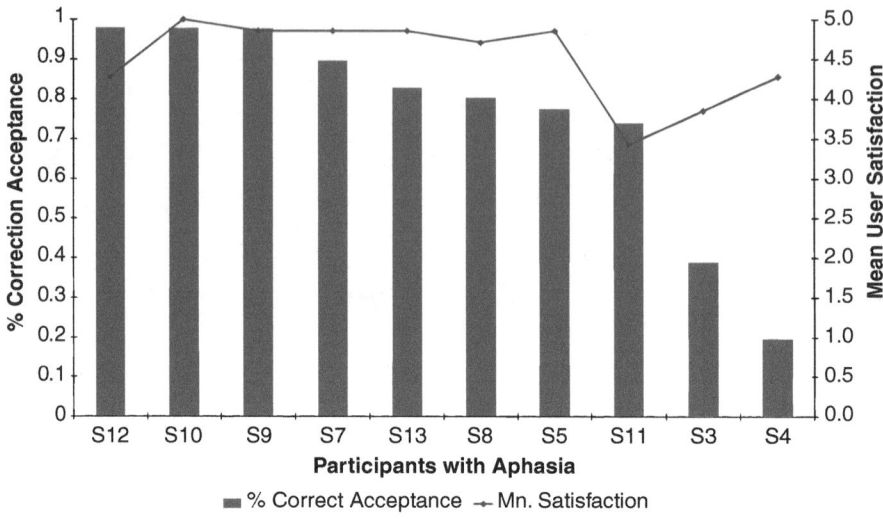

Fig. 8.6: Comparison of speech recognition accuracy and user satisfaction for 12 study participants with aphasia.

8.4 Conclusions

Our work with MTW-2 constitutes a preliminary step toward determining who is and who is not a good candidate for this type of technology and how a training procedure might be instituted for this population. We conclude that acceptable recognition accuracy can be achieved for most users, by adjusting the confidence sliders and/or phonological acceptance settings. For those who are still poorly recognized by the computer, a period of repeated use or formal adaptation training will likely allow the user and the recognizer to adapt to each other. If difficulty persists, an aphasia-friendly training protocol can be implemented. These findings support the work of Wade, Petheram and Cain (2001), who found that it is possible to bypass the linguistically complex standard training protocols in favor of training the software on specific vocabulary, and Abad et al. (2013) who used a calibration method to enable the recognizer to automatically adapt to the patient's speech characteristics. However, since some variation in performance remains, we cannot fully rely on the recognizer to provide feedback that is as accurate as feedback from a human scorer. Further, it remains to be determined whether speech recognition enhances the learning process and whether users will be able and willing to use this feature without the assistance of a speech-language pathologist or a computer coach. We have observed that when the recognizer does not understand the user, the user will, without instruction, speak louder or more carefully. This could prove beneficial for those wishing to improve their speech intelligibility and would be an important topic to explore experimentally.

8.5 Commercial programs using speech recognition for word retrieval deficits in aphasia

Currently, there are few commercial aphasia treatment programs that incorporate speech recognition or natural language understanding into their word retrieval training programs. Parrot software (www.parrotsoftware.com) and Constant Therapy (www.constanttherapy.com) are two popular programs that do use speech recognition in one or more of their treatment tasks, although neither report data on recognition accuracy or user satisfaction regarding this feature.

8.6 The challenge

There is a substantial body of evidence indicating that individuals with aphasia can learn to use computer-assisted treatments independently or with minimal support following training and that language skills can be enhanced and/or supported with the use of these programs. But there are many more evidence-based treatments that lend themselves to implementation with speech technology, and thus, there is much opportunity for a consortium of software designers, game developers, and users of aphasia software (people with aphasia, clinicians, and researchers) to collaborate and develop evidence-based products that are fun and easy to use.

Our experience with MTW suggests that it is possible to achieve good recognition accuracy with most users, but it took the support of a knowledgeable computer coach – and for those whose initial recognition accuracy was poor – a period of adaptation or aphasia-friendly training along with human support and encouragement. However, since this level of support is not always possible, SR software used in aphasia rehabilitation will need to be highly accurate with minimal or no training required. That is the challenge.

8.7 Moving beyond words

In Chapters 6–8, we have focused primarily on technology to help improve word retrieval. However, word retrieval treatment is only one aspect of an intervention program for people with aphasia. A complete intervention program needs to include ways to aid and support all aspects everyday communication (e.g. having conversations, creating e-mails, reading Facebook messages). In this regard, speech technology such as speech-to-text and text-to-speech (TTS) software can be very useful. While this technology has been discussed in great depth throughout the book, we conclude this chapter with a brief glimpse of how this technology is being used with individual with aphasia.

8.7.1 Speech-to-text/text-to-speech software

Since most smartphones and tablets now have speech recognition, a user can initiate a text message or search the Internet by speaking instead of typing. This feature can be extremely useful for individuals whose speaking skills are better than their writing skills, and some clinicians are bypassing traditional drill and practice software for universally designed programs that enable individuals with severe dysgraphia and milder verbal aphasias to use these systems to prepare and edit written communication. In a single subject study, Estes and Bloom (2011), trained a 65-year-old woman with conduction aphasia to use Dragon Naturally Speaking to improve her written production. Results revealed that, following intensive instruction, she was able to independently use the speech recognition program and her functional writing abilities had improved.

In our aphasia center (MossRehab Aphasia Center), we have also observed how speech technology reduces barriers for individuals with aphasia whose reading and writing are severely limited. One tech-savvy client with aphasia successfully uses his smartphone's speech technology to search the Internet and send text and e-mail messages. While we continue to work on improving his reading and writing skills, speech-to-text technology allows him to function independently in his everyday life. Unfortunately, not all individuals with aphasia are tech-savvy prior to aphasia. We have found that direct training and tech support are essential parts of any intervention program that incorporates technology.

Similarly, TTS programs such as WordQ (2015) will not only speak the written text but will also provide assistance with word prediction. Some reading and writing programs can be set to enlarge and highlight words as the computer reads them. This might help with reading comprehension and oral reading because the user will see and hear the words as he is reading. TTS might also help correct writing errors because the user will hear the word he is typing as well as see it, thus heightening his ability to monitor errors. Creative clinicians can develop thematic-based treatment based on topics of interest to the user (e.g. sports, travel, dining) and create vocabulary, and scripts for practice and/or playback. Functional phrases and word lists can be typed in by a therapist or family member and then practiced by having the screen-reading program read the word or sentence aloud and teaching the patient to repeat it.

We have used WordQ with a patient (Mr. P.) with severe Wernicke's aphasia who was charged with delivering an annual report to his board of directors. The client worked with his clinician to develop the talking points and the clinician edited the language and grammar, turning the speech into short, but meaningful points that Mr. P. could rehearse both in therapy and at home on his computer. After weeks of intensive practice, playing, and repeating each talking point, Mr. P. successfully spoke the entire speech without the use of the text reader.

We have also used TTS to enable people with severe aphasia to communicate messages they are unable to speak. Speak It!, an app for the iPad and Android device enables users (or communication partners) to type in a phrase or message for the person with aphasia to play back at another time. TTS may also be useful for people with aphasia whose slowed reading rate affects functional use of reading or when time limitations are present.

There is a paucity of research in this area, but at least two published studies have reported beneficial effects following training on computer software that supports writing with word prediction, spell check (Behrns, Hartelius & Wenfelin 2009) and a talking word processor (King & Hux 1995). Text simplification programs may also be useful for individuals with aphasia who typically also have acquired reading impairments (dyslexia) (Devlin & Unthank 2006).

Some commercial programs use speech technology to allow users to record and play back their speech. This feature can provide valuable assistance in facilitating self-monitoring. Locutour (Learning Fundamental: www.learningfundamentals.com), for example, has a series of articulation programs that allow the user to see a picture, hear a word, phrase, or sentence, and then record the same utterance, play back their attempts to repeat, or name and compare their response to the model. Recording and playing back a recently recorded utterance can also help a user keep his utterance in memory, an issue that is addressed by a unique software program called SentenceShaper®, which will be discussed in the following chapter, by Marcia Linebarger.

8.7.2 Role of the speech-language pathologist

To best guide their clients, speech-language pathologists now have a responsibility to be familiar with available technology and how to match the technology to the needs of each client with whom they work. Keeping up with this rapidly advancing field is quite challenging, and some aphasia centers now employ technology experts as part of their team to support both themselves and their clients. While the speech-language pathologist is well suited to evaluate and recommend which technology to use and/or to guide the user in how best to use the technology, the learning curve for understanding new software may be too steep for the time they have in their daily practice. This is an issue that will need to be addressed.

References

Abad, A., Pompili, A., Costa, Trancoso, I. Fonseca, J., Leal, G., Farrajota, L., Martins, I. P. (2013). Automatic word naming recognition for an on-line aphasia treatment system. *Computer Speech & Language 27*, 1235–1348.

Behrns, I., Hartelius, L. & Wengelin, A. (2009). Aphasia and computerized writing aid supported treatment. *Aphasiology 23*, 1276–1294.

Devlin, S. & Unthank, G. (2006). Helping aphasic people process online information. In *Proceeding of the 8th International ACM SIGACCESS Conference on Computers and Accessibility* (pp. 225–226).

Estes, C. & Bloom, R. (2011). Using voice recognition software to treat dysgraphia in a patient with conduction aphasia. *Aphasiology 25*, 366–385.

Fink, R. B., Brecher, A., Montgomery, M. & Schwarz, M. F. (2001) MossTalk Words (Computer software manual). Philadelphia: Albert Einstein Healthcare Network.

Fink, R. B. & Dahl, D. (2012). *MossTalk Words-2: Can a computer understand and respond appropriately to aphasic speakers?* Presented at Topics in Rehabilitation Science, Philadelphia, PA, USA.

Fink, R. B., Brecher, A., Schwartz, M. F. & Robey, R. R. (2002). A computer implemented protocol for treatment of naming disorders: Evaluation of clinician-guided and partially self-guided instruction. *Aphasiology 16*, 1061–1086.

Fink, R. B., Schwartz, M. & Dahl, D. A. (2009). Using speech recognition for speech therapy: MossTalkWords 2.0. Poster presentation at the Annual Meeting of the *American Speech-Language-Hearing Association*, November 21–22, New Orleans, LA, USA.

Howard, D., Patterson, K., Franklin, S., Orchard-Lisle, V. & Morton, J. (1985a). The facilitation of picture naming in aphasia. *Cognitive Neuropsychology 2*, 49–80.

Howard, D., Patterson, K., Franklin, S., Orchard-Lisle, V. & Morton, J. (1985b). Treatment of word retrieval deficits in aphasia: A comparison of 2 therapy methods. *Brain 108*, 817–829.

Jokel, R., Cupit, J., Rochon, E. & Graham, N. (2007). Errorless re-training in semantic dementia using MossTalk words. *Brain and Language 103*, 205–206.

Jokel, R., Cupit, J., Rochon, E. & Leonard, C. (2006). Computer-based intervention for anomia in progressive aphasia. *Brain and Language 99*, 149–150.

Jokel, R., Cupit, J., Rochon, E. & Leonard, C. (2009). Relearning lost vocabulary in nonfluent progressive aphasia with MossTalk words. *Aphasiology 23*, 175–191.

Jokel, R., Rochon, E. & Anderson, N. D. (2010). Errorless learning of computer-generated words in a patient with semantic dementia. *Neuropsychological Rehabilitation 20*, 16–41.

King, J. M. & Hux, K. (1995). Intervention using talking word processing software: An aphasia case study. *Augmentative and Alternative Communication Journal, 11*, 187–192.

Linebaugh, C. & Lehner, L. (1977). *Cueing hierarchies and word retrieval: A treatment program.* Minneapolis, MN: BRK Publishers.

Ramsberger, G. & Marie, B. (2005). Self-administered MossTalk Words: A single subject design comparing treatment intensity replicated in three cases. *Brain and Language, 95*, 207–208.

Ramsberger, G. & Marie, B. (2007). Self-administered cued naming therapy: A single-participant investigation of a computer-based therapy program replicated in four cases. *American Journal of Speech-Language Pathology 16*, 343–358.

Raymer, A., Carwile, K., Matthews, M., Johnson, T. & Todd, T. (2009). MossTalk training for word retrieval: Generalization across semantic categories. Presented at *39th Clinical Aphasiology Conference*, Keystone, CO, USA.

Raymer, A., Kohen, F. & Saffel, D. (2006). Computerized training for impairments of word comprehension and retrieval in aphasia. *Aphasiology 20*, 257–268.

Sobel, P., Fink, R. & Schwartz, M. F. (2000). The impact of computer-assisted aphasia therapy in the outpatient aphasia clinical setting: Final Report on a study funded by the McLean Contributionship. Unpublished manuscript available from the authors.

Thompson, C. K., Raymer, A. M. & Le Grand, H. R. (1991). Effects of phonologically based treatment on aphasic naming deficits: A model-driven approach. *Clinical Aphasiology 20*, 239–262.

Wade, J., Petheram, B. & Cain, R. (2001). Voice recognition and aphasia: Can computers understand aphasic speech? *Disability Rehabilitation, 23*, 604–613.

WordQ. (2015). Retrieved from http://www.synapseadaptive.com/quillsoft/WQ/wordq_features.htm

Marcia Linebarger

9 Speech technology for aphasic sentence production disorders

Abstract: Chapter 9 focuses on language production at the sentence level and beyond, looking at the role of speech technology in treatment and at the use of speech technology to aid communication and decrease social isolation. The chapter begins with a discussion of non-fluent aphasia, and the theory behind current approaches to treatment. Then, as elsewhere in this book, we share our own experiences in developing and studying speech-based software for aphasia. This chapter describes two programs developed by the author and colleagues. One of these programs used speech recognition and natural language understanding to provide feedback about the correctness of spoken picture descriptions. The other program, SentenceShaper®, simply records the user's speech, but provides a visual interface which allows the user to build small fragments of speech into larger utterances. The research on both programs is reviewed briefly. The chapter concludes with a survey of other currently available speech technology applications that can support language production in aphasia as treatment tools, communication aids, or other resources to improve language and quality of life for people with aphasia.

9.1 Background: language production in non-fluent aphasia

The speech of a person with non-fluent aphasia can easily strike the listener as a catastrophic loss of grammatical abilities. For example, below is the speech of a woman with agrammatic aphasia. She is describing a scene in a wordless video. In this scene, a boy walks into a fish store while the owner is hitting a fish with a mallet. The boy reaches for the fish, and his hand is hit by the mallet. Her description:

> "A fish! Ah, water" and ... uh mmm and attendant, 'here' and bumped his head. "Oh boy, oh my hand, my hand, my hand."

Clearly in short supply are sentences, verbs (one, compared with the four verbs we used in our summary of the event, above), and prepositions (none, compared with four in our version). The scarcity of such relational elements is widely noted in the aphasia literature. Individuals with this speech pattern, termed agrammatism, often show a comprehension impairment ('asyntactic comprehension') that appears to reflect a similar insensitivity to grammatical structure.

Despite the impression of a central loss of grammatical ability, most aphasiologists have moved away from accounts of this speech pattern as reflecting an outright loss of linguistic knowledge. One compelling source of evidence is the fact that many people with agrammatic aphasia and asyntactic comprehension demonstrate near-normal sensitivity to grammatical structure in grammaticality judgment tasks (Friederici 1982; Linebarger, Schwartz & Saffran 1983; Shankweiler, Crain, Gorrell & Tuller 1988; Wulfeck, Bates & Capasso 1991). A complementary argument against the view of agrammatism as reflecting loss of grammatical knowledge is that neurologically unimpaired individuals can show very similar comprehension impairments (i.e. asyntactic comprehension) when processing demands are increased, as in dual-task paradigms (Miyake, Carpenter & Just 1994; Blackwell & Bates 1995). If the asyntactic comprehension pattern associated with agrammatic aphasia can be induced in unimpaired individuals by increasing their processing load, then it need not be taken as an indication that grammatical knowledge has been lost in aphasia.

9.1.1 Explanations

But if agrammatic speakers have not, so to speak, simply forgotten the rules of their language, what is the reason for the fragmented speech we saw above, consisting largely of nouns not linked together by verbs, prepositions, or other relational words? Factors such as the following have been proposed.

9.1.1.1 Pathologically reduced short-term/working memory or resource diminution

What we will loosely term "processing limitations" could result in failure to maintain sentence elements long enough to build them into larger structures for comprehension (Miyake, Carpenter & Just 1994; Blackwell & Bates 1995; Caplan & Waters 1995) or production (Kolk & Heeschen 1992; Kolk 1995) and could result in the kind of fragmented agrammatic production we saw above. Strong supporting evidence for this view has also come from markedly improved sentence production on SentenceShaper®, a software program that provides memory support. This will be discussed below.

9.1.1.2 Weak activation of linguistic elements
Knowledge is not, of course, all or nothing. Words and structures may be weakly present, enough for recognition but not for production. The evidence for syntactic priming in agrammatic speakers (Saffran & Martin 1990; Hartsuiker & Kolk 1998) suggests that the knowledge has not been lost, but may need to be primed in order to be used for production. In these studies, agrammatic participants described pictures using syntactic structures normally absent from their speech immediately following exposure to, and repetition of, sentences containing the same structures.

9.1.1.3 Difficulty with "thinking for speaking"
Problems at the interface between the conceptual and the linguistic (Levelt 1989; Slobin 1996; Marshall & Cairns 2005; Dipper, Black & Bryan 2005) have also been suggested. Consider an event such as the fish store fiasco described above. To convert it into the series of sentences above, we have to select the most important details (ignoring, for example, that the boy has red hair or the fishmonger is bald, not talking about the boy's motivation in reaching for the fish or the fact that it is flopping around) and carve up the story into a series of sentence-size events. This process is intimately linked to our knowledge of the words available in English, so both linguistic and conceptual information must be accessed at the same time, to create representations which (in the words of Marshall and Cairns) "have propositional structure, encode perspective, and are tuned to the target language of the speaker" (Marshall & Cairns 2005).

Failure to create such a representation would prevent the speaker from coming up with words and/or structuring them correctly.

We need not think of impaired "thinking for speaking" as a third, distinct, mechanism, since the combination of limited memory space and weak activation of linguistic information could cause a disruption at this stage of language production. On this account, the impaired verb retrieval observed in non-fluent aphasia is a subcase of this problem: since verbs describe a particular relationship among different entities, the speaker must be able to maintain a representation of the event and link it to the words of his language. Impaired working memory could make it hard to keep the potential predicates and arguments alive in memory, and weak activation of linguistic elements could make it hard to provide an appropriate verb to guide this representation. In contrast, retrieval of concrete, imageable nouns does not require the maintenance of such a complex representation.

The "mapping hypothesis" (Linebarger et al. 1993; Schwartz, Linebarger & Saffran 1985), which proposed that agrammatism reflects difficulty in mapping syntactic structure onto meaning as opposed to an inability to compute syntactic structure in and of itself, belongs to this same family of explanations because it points to a problem at the interface of grammar and meaning. The mapping hypothesis targets the relationship between grammatical roles like subject and semantic roles like agent.

The challenge of thinking for speaking is most striking in the task of narrative production. For most aphasic speakers, multi-sentence narratives describing complex events are far more difficult to create than single-picture descriptions (e.g. Lesser 1989; Mitchum & Berndt 1994; Weinrich, Shelton, McCall & Cox 1997). Improved narrative production is an important goal of treatment, because it is strongly linked to functionally relevant measures (e.g. Frattali, Thompson, Holland, Wohl & Ferketic 1995; Doyle, Tsironas, Goda & Kalinyak 1996; Ross & Wertz 1999; Jacobs 2001). As Kempler and Goral (2011) observe:

> telling personal narratives require[s] participants to generate multiple linked utterances without visual support of pictures. Personal narratives are an appropriate assessment of functional language use as they occur in many discourse contexts from reporting daily events to telling jokes and stories, and can contribute to an individual's ability to understand life experiences, present oneself to others, and participate in various communal and communicative events. Indeed, it might be argued that one ultimate goal of aphasia treatment is functional production and comprehension of narratives.

Unfortunately, treatment gains have rarely generalized from more constrained laboratory tasks such as single-picture description to the production of connected speech (see, e.g. Berndt & Mitchum 1995). Therefore, treatments that result in improved narrative production are of particular interest.

9.1.2 Approaches to treating sentence production in non-fluent aphasia

What are the implications of these hypotheses for the treatment of language production disorders? One general conclusion is that people with non-fluent aphasia do not need to be re-taught their language in the way we might teach a foreign language to a brand new speaker. The language is still there, albeit weakly activated, and rendered still more inaccessible by a limited memory buffer in which to combine words into sentences. And providing external correction of errors may be less important than it would be for, e.g., second-language learners.

One two-pronged strategy consistent with the view above is this: use drill exercises to raise the activation level of words and structures, but also engage the speaker in tasks that require thinking for speaking – that is, tasks that require one to access language from the "back end", at the point at which conceptual representations are propositionalized and linked to specific words and structures. In practice, many clinicians do incorporate both approaches to treatment.

9.1.2.1 Drill/practice exercises to increase activation of particular items or structures

In this category, we include treatments that involve the priming (through exposure and/or repetition) of particular structures; or, as in Syntax Stimulation (Helm-Estabrooks 1981), to a wide variety of structures. Similarly, drilling on individual words should help to make them more available for sentence production.

However, it has generally been the case that such exercises alone do not generalize beyond single-picture description, sometimes only for the trained items. One explanation is that they rarely train thinking for speaking. A picture description task does a great deal of the work of event processing: it presents the user with one event and clearly depicted participants, often normed beforehand to make sure that it elicits a specific sentence. In addition, it may be that the limited memory buffer simply prevents the speaker from practicing the actual process of sentence construction, even in drills targeting full sentences. Repetition drills, for example, may draw upon auditory verbal memory rather than upon normal sentence construction processes; in repeating "The man is walking the dog", a participant may in actuality be repeating something more like a single word ("themaniswalkingthedog").

This is not to say that such drills are not important. There may be tremendous impact on social functioning to be able to produce even fixed social phrases or scripts, as emphasized in Script Training (Cherney, Halper, Holland & Cole 2008); and drill-based activation of words and structures is almost certainly a necessary component of treatment for aphasic sentence production disorders.

9.1.2.2 Treatments to improve thinking for speaking

Treatments in this category can be seen along a continuum of informational open-endedness.

At one end are tasks in which the user practices describing an unambiguous event, usually represented in a picture. Both client and clinician are familiar with the event, so no novel information is conveyed. The clinician guides the user through selection of the important building blocks of the sentence, such as the verb, and its arguments. Some of the "event parsing" exercises of Marshall and colleagues start at the single-picture level. Similarly, mapping therapy (Byng 1988; Byng, Nickels & Black 1994; Schwartz, Saffran, Fink, Myers & Martin 1994; Rochon, Laird, Bose & Scofield 2005) trains the speaker to focus upon specific relationships (pick a verb and say who is doing what to whom), which – in addition to its core goal of providing practice in making specific associations between grammatical and thematic roles – may also help with event parsing and cutting down the search space of what to verbalize. A similar focus on extracting verb and arguments is provided by treatments like Sentactics® (Thompson, Choy, Holland & Cole 2010), which involve probing for verb, agent, and theme in active sentences and their object-relative counterparts. In all these cases, a stimulus is presented to the speaker to practice strategies for expressing the most conceptually and/or grammatically important actions and actors.

Moving further down the continuum toward greater open-endedness are treatments like VNeST (Emonds, Nadeau & Kiran 2009), which focuses upon activating not just the verb but also sets of subject and object arguments. The protocol involves training specific verbs (e.g. "measure") by eliciting appropriate arguments (for example, "carpenter" and "stairs"). Those who cannot produce arguments on their own are offered choices among appropriate and inappropriate arguments, but the goal is for the client to produce a variety of arguments independently. This differs from mapping therapy and Sentactics because rather than training the user to search efficiently for the main participants in an already depicted action, it requires the user to create new propositions, constrained by the semantics and syntax of the training verb.

The most open-ended "thinking for speaking" task would seem to be the creation of multi-sentence narratives, whether retellings of story-level videos or the creation of personal narratives. This requires the speaker to identify important participants and actions, select a perspective, and decompose a complex story into segments compatible with the speaker's language. Two case studies focusing upon narrative production tasks (Marshall, Pring & Chiat 1998; Peach & Wong 2004) resulted in impressive gains in narrative production.

Unfortunately, a significant problem with narrative production as a treatment task – or even as an assessment measure – is that processing limitations and word-finding problems can make it virtually impossible to accomplish without intensive clinician support. In the Peach and Wong study (2004), for example, the clinician wrote down everything that the participant said, read it back to her, incorporated any corrections/additions, and so forth. In the narrative production tasks of Marshall and colleagues, there was considerable clinician involvement in helping the participant to, so to speak, bite off manageable chunks of the story and turn them into sentences.

Now we will ask – can speech technology help to deliver the two general types of sentence production treatment described above? That is, can it help to provide drilling, to activate sentence structures, and also support treatments that target thinking for speaking?

9.2 Scope of the term "speech technology"

We will use the term "speech technology" here to refer to computer software that takes as input the user's spoken utterances and facilitates speech therapy, or simply communication, in people with aphasia. There are basically three things that a program can do in this context:
- Analyze the user's speech, by turning it into text and possibly determining its intended meaning;
- Record the user's speech;
- Transmit the user's speech to others.

Below we will review software that performs one or more of these operations, and discuss how it can improve language and communication in non-fluent aphasia.

9.3 A tale of two programs

As noted in the introduction, one goal of this book is to share the authors' own experiences developing speech technology applications for people with language disorders. Therefore, we will begin by describing in detail two programs that were developed and/or studied by one of the authors (M.L.) and colleagues. By and large, these programs embody each of the two approaches to treatment outlined above (drilling versus thinking for speaking) and use different kinds of speech technology. The first program was designed to implement a sentence production drill exercise focused upon sentences with prepositions, with the goal of activating prepositional words and structures. The second program was designed to implement what we will refer to loosely as a "thinking for speaking" approach to treatment, by supporting more open-ended speech, including narrative production.

9.3.1 The "TS": using speech technology for sentence production drills

In the late 1990s, we developed and studied a treatment program for agrammatic aphasia (Linebarger, Schwartz & Kohn 2001; Linebarger & Romania 2007) which incorporated speech recognition and natural language understanding. The program – referred to here as the "TS", short for Therapy System – displayed a picture for the user to describe in a spoken sentence. Target sentences contained prepositional phrases, first in simple locative assertions ("The bird is on the cup"), then in subject-verb-object sentences with locative prepositional phrases ("The dog is licking the baby under the chair"), and finally in subject-verb-object sentences with prepositional phrases indicating direction ("The clown is pushing the dancer into the pool").

Because the TS was designed to implement some features of mapping therapy, the focus was on using grammatical word order to signal thematic roles. The scenarios were all reversible, in the sense that each sentence contained at least two nouns that would be semantically appropriate as subject or object (direct or prepositional).

Each trial began with the program asking the user to say aloud the verb and/ or preposition. Word-finding help was available from icons on the screen, and the program offered feedback about correctness. Then the user was asked to "say the whole sentence". When the user finished speaking, the program analyzed the sentence – incorporating both speech recognition, which created a text transcript of the spoken sentence, and natural language understanding, which provided a representation of thematic roles based upon this text transcript.[1] Because it recovered the text and "meaning" of the user's sentence, the program was able to provide detailed feedback about correctness. It was specifically designed to catch word order errors (for example, reversing subject and object) or omissions (for example, leaving out the object, as in "The clown is pushing into the pool"). The program incorporated speech grammars, which permitted a variety of synonyms (for example, users could say, "woman" instead of "dancer").

The feedback was both visual and auditory. Missing or incorrectly ordered elements were decolorized, and the program provided feedback such as, "Yes, you are right, the clown is pushing someone into the pool. Who is he pushing?" Correct responses were rewarded with musical feedback. In addition, the program tracked usage and correctness, providing feedback to the user at the end of each session.

The speech recognition was imperfect. Some recognition errors were not critical to the purpose of the program: for example, grammatical function words were often ignored or recognized incorrectly. Therefore, even if the user said, "the clown is pushing the dancer into the pool", the speech recognizer might hear this as "clown pushing dancer into pool". We compensated for this by designing the speech grammars so that they accepted, and analyzed, such sentences rather than trying to correct them. That is, missing articles and auxiliaries were ignored because the focus of the program was on the roles expressed by subject, object, and prepositional object.[2]

---

[1] To avoid confusing or distracting the user, the TS did not display the actual text of the speech recognizer's hypothesis.

[2] Of course, if the user were to utter a passive sentence such as "The dancer is pushed by the clown", the speech recognizer's tendency to ignore function words and morphology could lead to an incorrect hypothesis, "The dancer pushed the clown". But the passive, a notoriously difficult structure for this population, was virtually never used by participants in the study.

Despite these measures, the speech recognition was sometimes incorrect in ways that did matter, such as hearing the wrong preposition. This was, of course, frustrating to users. For that reason, we added a button allowing users to play back a recording of what they had actually said. This allowed them to decide for themselves whether negative feedback from the program was justified.

The program also provided word-finding support: clicking a pictured object on the screen caused the program to play its name; verbs and prepositions were available by clicking icons.

Shown in Fig. 9.1 is a TS screen in the "locative assertions" module, for the target sentence "The bird is behind the cup". The two buttons at the bottom turn the speech recognizer on and off. Touching the "P" icon plays the preposition "behind". Touching the bird and glass images plays those nouns. The arrow pointing to the bird instructs the user to start with that noun.

In summary, the TS provided a relatively standard drill exercise (picture description of the same structure repeated over many trials) enhanced with feedback about correctness made possible by speech recognition and natural language understanding.

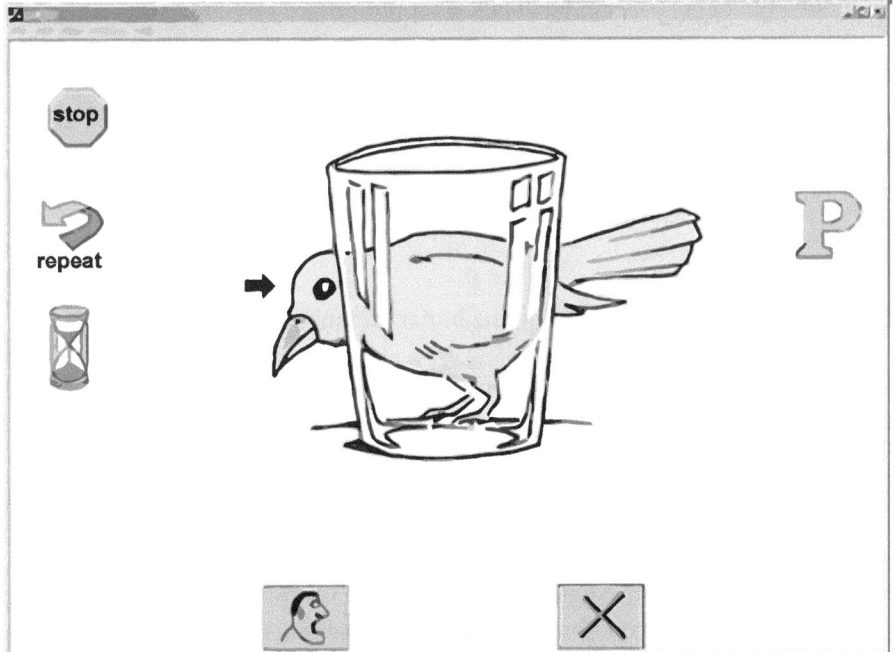

Fig. 9.1: Therapy System (TS): screen in the Locative Assertions module.

An exploratory study with the TS (Linebarger et al. 2001) reported that home use of the program increased accurate production of the trained prepositions and structures for five participants with agrammatic aphasia. Results were most marked for the two least impaired participants. For example, participant JT's production of correct picture descriptions for simple locative assertions increased (for untrained stimuli) from 48% to 96% correct; participant JW increased from 33% to 90%.

So, was speech technology worthwhile in this program? Although the technology did not provide any functionality that would not have been available from a clinician, it did provide (1) the opportunity to practice independently at home, (2) feedback about correctness, and (3) a sense of accomplishment from having the computer understand their speech.

Regarding independence, any computerized treatment program offers that opportunity, and many commercially available programs provide drill on different sentence types.

As for feedback, it remains an open question whether the program's detailed feedback about errors and verb/preposition or argument omissions was helpful in retraining the structure, given the evidence that even those who speak ungrammatically may be able to detect errors in a grammaticality judgment task. More generally, the importance of feedback is an unresolved issue in aphasia therapy (e.g. Breitenstein, Kamping, Jansen, Schomacher & Knecht 2004 reported that feedback was not crucial in a word learning task for aphasia).

Finally, what about motivation? It was our subjective impression that the feedback afforded by speech technology made the program more interesting to participants, but there are no data that speak to this point, for the TS or other sentence-level aphasia software.

9.3.2 SentenceShaper: enlarging the buffer for language

Despite this fairly successful deployment of speech technology, observing the study participants using the TS described suggested a very different approach. Two observations in particular were striking:

- Impact of memory decay: Observing use of the TS's word-finding support demonstrated vividly the impact of memory limitations on sentence production. Users might click the screen to get help with the word "clown", then struggle for a long time to retrieve the verb "push", or simply get it by clicking the verb icon. But then, when they went to say the whole sentence, they would have to re-retrieve the word "clown", by which time the verb icon might have to be re-clicked again.

– Need for self-monitoring: Another program feature turned out to be quite revealing. Recall that we had added a button to let users replay their own recorded utterances, primarily as a way to counteract the frustration caused by a speech recognizer malfunction. But we observed that the act of self-replay was very helpful. Typically, users were mystified by the program's corrections and would replay their own utterance primarily to confirm their assumption that the speech recognizer had erred. But then, quite often, there would be an "aha!" moment, as they listened to their own utterance and compared it to the picture. The program's correction, while it may have alerted them that something was wrong, did not really "take" until they actually listened to what they themselves had said. This suggested that self-monitoring may be at least as important as feedback from the software.

These two observations arising from the TS led to the development of SentenceShaper[3] (Linebarger, Schwartz, Romania, Kohn & Stephens 2000; SentenceShaper 2015; Linebarger & Romania 2000), a program designed to help users retain in memory those words that they can retrieve, and to help them build their recorded utterances into more complex structures than they would otherwise be able to produce.

9.3.2.1 How the program works

SentenceShaper combines a sound recorder with a visual interface that lets the user combine small chunks of recorded speech into sentences and full messages.

The user records a chunk of speech – a word, a phrase, etc. – by clicking a button on the screen. Each recording gets linked to a small crystal icon. Whenever the user clicks that crystal icon, it will play back the recording. This combination of a recording and a crystal icon is called a "snippet". Figure 9.2 shows a snippet that the user has just recorded, using the Microphone Button at the bottom of the screen. (The contents of this chunk of recorded speech are indicated in the figure with text, but the program itself does not display the text of users' utterances, a point to which we return below.) Let us say that the user is trying to talk about a boy eating an apple and that the first word that has come to his mind is "apple".

When the user clicks that snippet, it will replay his recording, "apple". Although this is not a good agent for the act of eating and is therefore unlikely to be the first word of the sentence, recording it as soon as it comes to mind is a way

---

3 SentenceShaper was referred to as "CS" (Communication System) in research studies publis-hed before 2006.

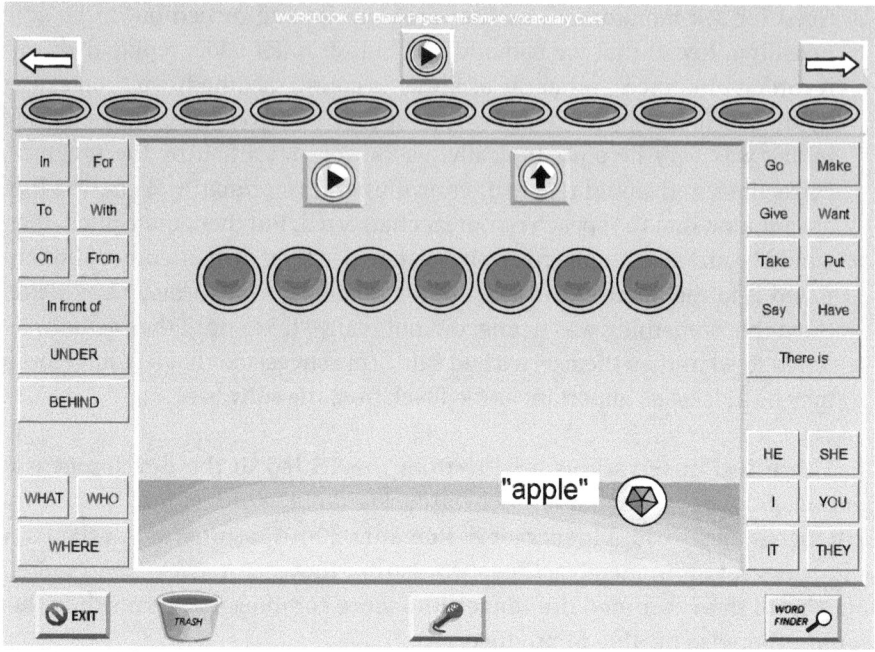

Fig. 9.2: SentenceShaper: snippet in the Work Area.

to keep it in memory. The user will not have to keep re-retrieving this word, as we observed participants doing with the TS.

When a snippet is first recorded, it appears in the Work Area, at the bottom of the screen near the Microphone Button. Snippets appear in random order, associated with random abstract icons. Figure 9.3 shows the Work Area with two more snippets, "eat" and "the boy".

Snippets are combined into sentences by dragging them to a different area of the screen, the Sentence Row, where they can be ordered, re-ordered, played in order, removed from the Sentence Row, or supplemented with additional snippets. Figure 9.4 shows these snippets ordered in the Sentence Row, but in an implausible order (since apples rarely eat boys).

An important part of using the program is self-monitoring. Material in the Sentence Row can be replayed by clicking the "play button" on the upper left of the Sentence Row. When our user replays the entire sequence, he may well notice the misordering and correct it by rearranging the snippets. The corrected version is shown in Fig. 9.5.

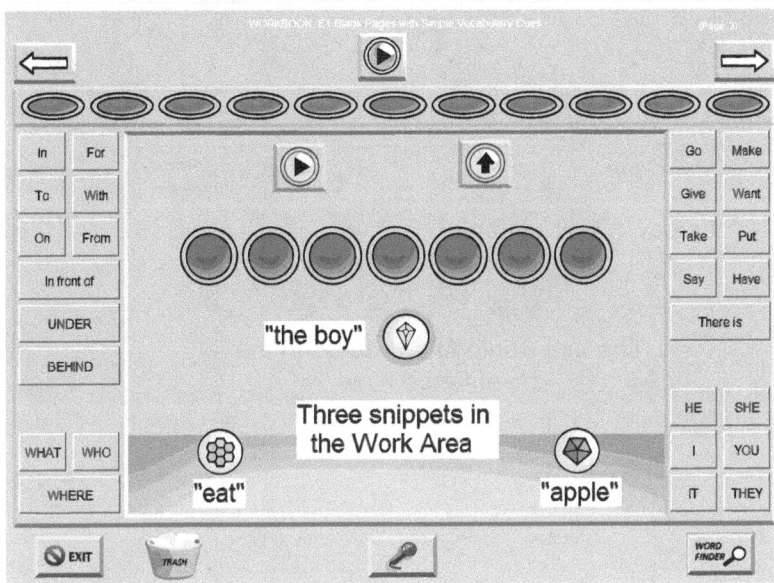

Fig. 9.3: SentenceShaper: three snippets in the Work Area.

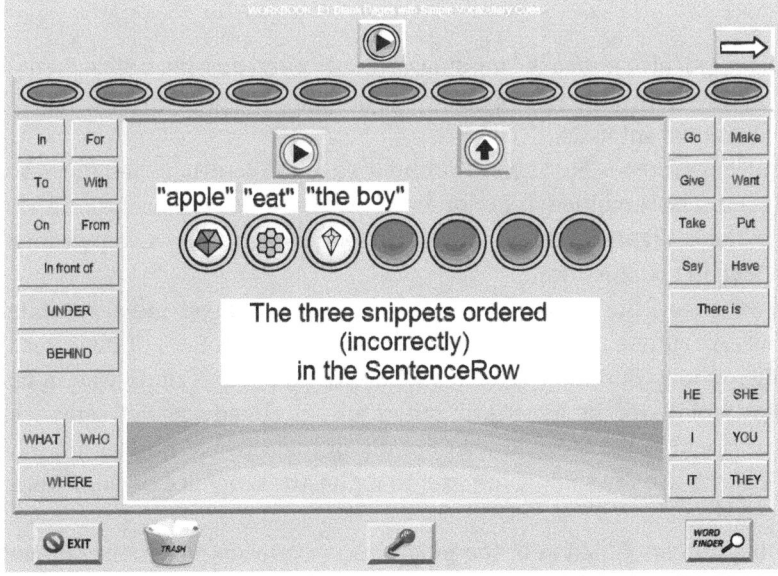

Fig. 9.4: SentenceShaper: snippets in the Sentence Row, ordered incorrectly.

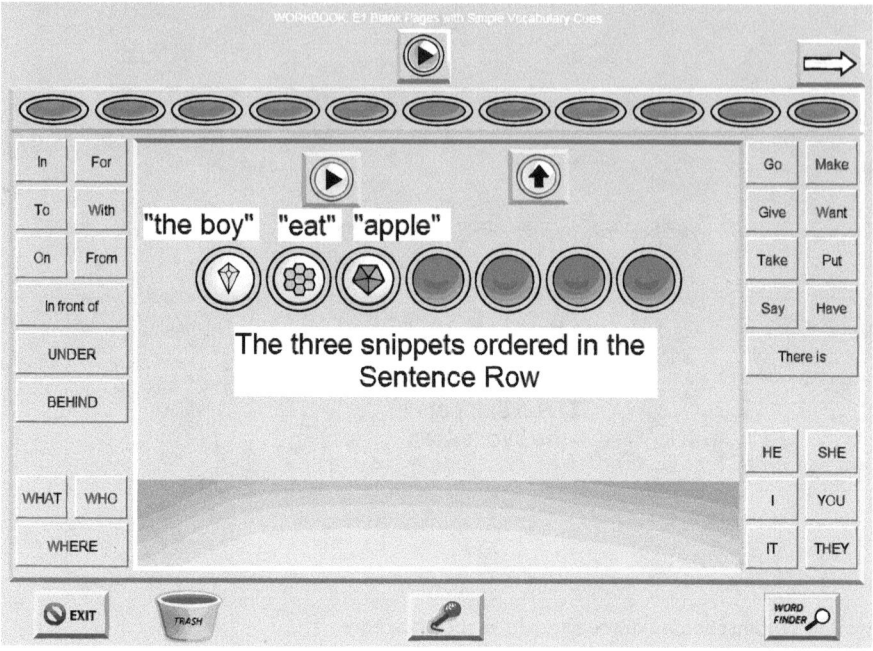

Fig. 9.5: Snippets in the Sentence Row, ordered correctly.

The user might also notice the missing verb suffix and missing article; in that case, he would re-record the existing snippets or repair the ungrammaticality by recording additional snippets.

A completed sentence is added to a third area of the screen, called the Story Row, where it can be combined it with other sentences to create speeches, stories, or other messages. Figure 9.6 shows this same sequence of snippets represented by a single icon in the Story Row.

Figure 9.7 shows the SentenceShaper screen with a larger message under construction. Six snippets appear in the Work Area at the bottom of the screen, near the Microphone Button; a sentence with four snippets is underway in the Sentence Row (middle of the screen), and there are two already-created sentences (purple oval icons) in the Story Row at the top of the screen. The Play Buttons above each of the two rows allow the user to replay the sequence of elements in that row.

While the primary function of the program is to provide processing support and facilitate self-monitoring, SentenceShaper also provides word-finding support. Along the side of the screen there are, optionally, Vocabulary Cue Buttons with text words or labels displayed. Clicking a button plays the word, and the user

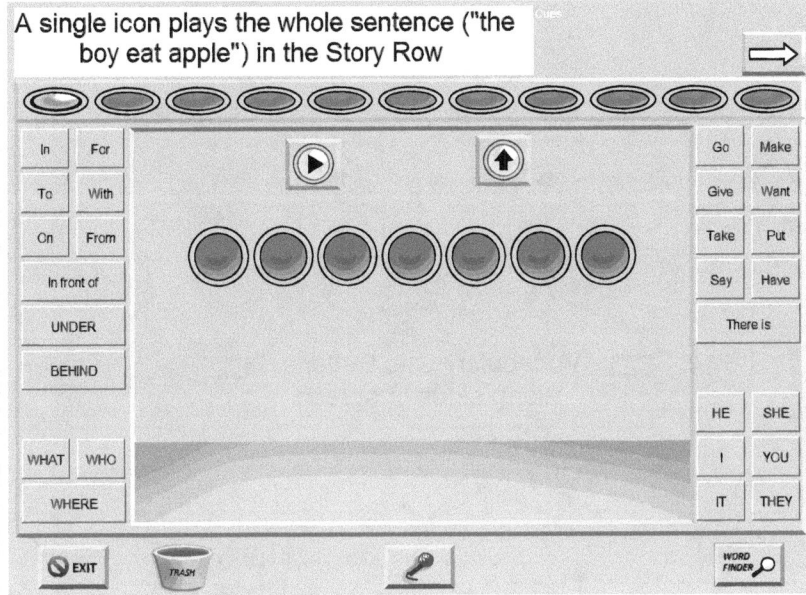

Fig. 9.6: Icon in the Sentence Row.

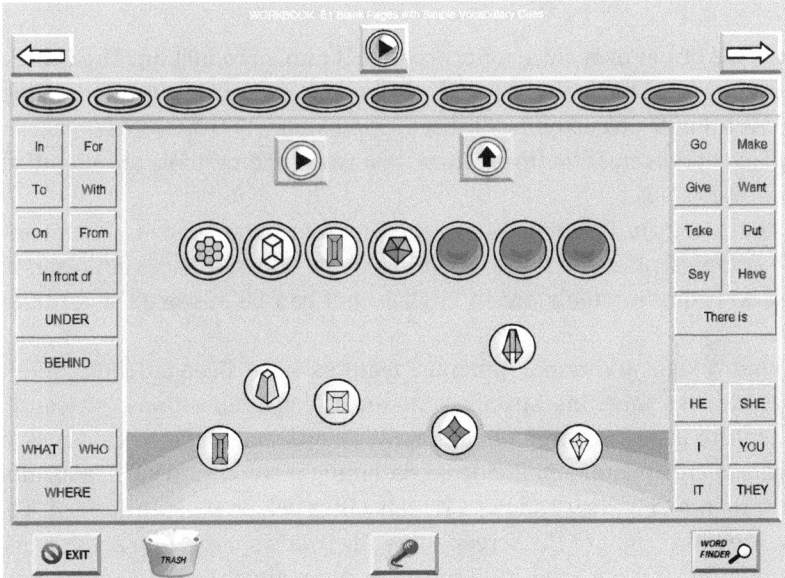

Fig. 9.7: Icons in the Story Row, Sentence Row, and Work Area.

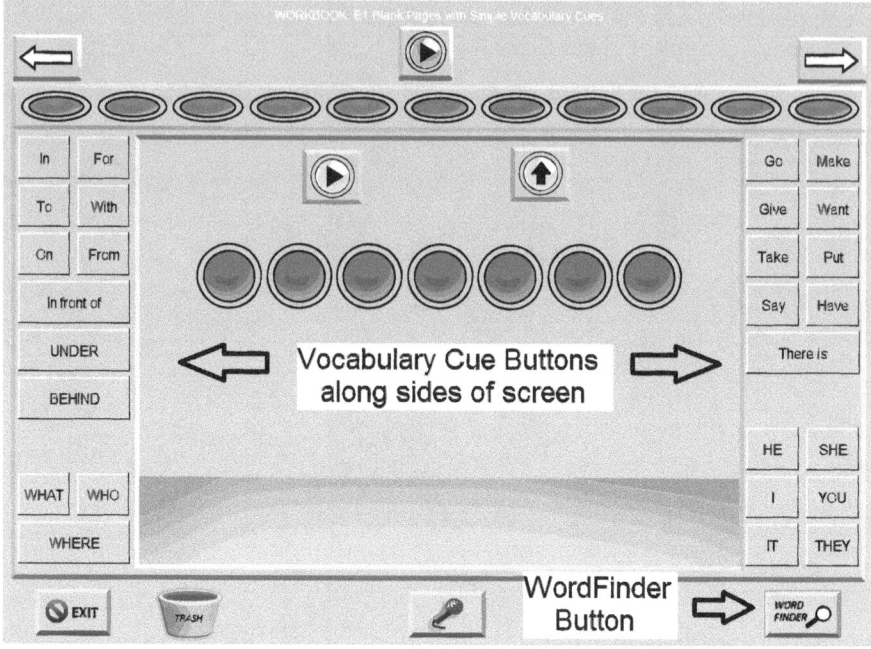

Fig. 9.8: Word-finding tools.

records it in his or her own voice to incorporate it into a production. The content of these buttons is customizable. There is also a more extensive word-finding tool called the WordFinder, a customizable list of approximately 1100 words organized along syntactic and semantic lines. These two word-finding tools are identified with arrows in Fig. 9.8.

Note that the core functionality of the program is language-independent: recording snippets of speech and grouping them into sentences and messages. These word-finding tools are in English, but can be customized for other languages.

In recent years, additional program features have been added: built-in therapy workbooks targeting specific structures (e.g. prepositions, "because" clauses); tools to insert personal photographs; an optional text area on the main screen; tools to create and e-mail videos containing pictures and speech created within the program. Figure 9.9 shows a screen with a personal picture added. The button on the lower right of the screen turns the user's speech into a video and opens a simplified interface to e-mail the video as an attachment to one or more of the user's contacts.

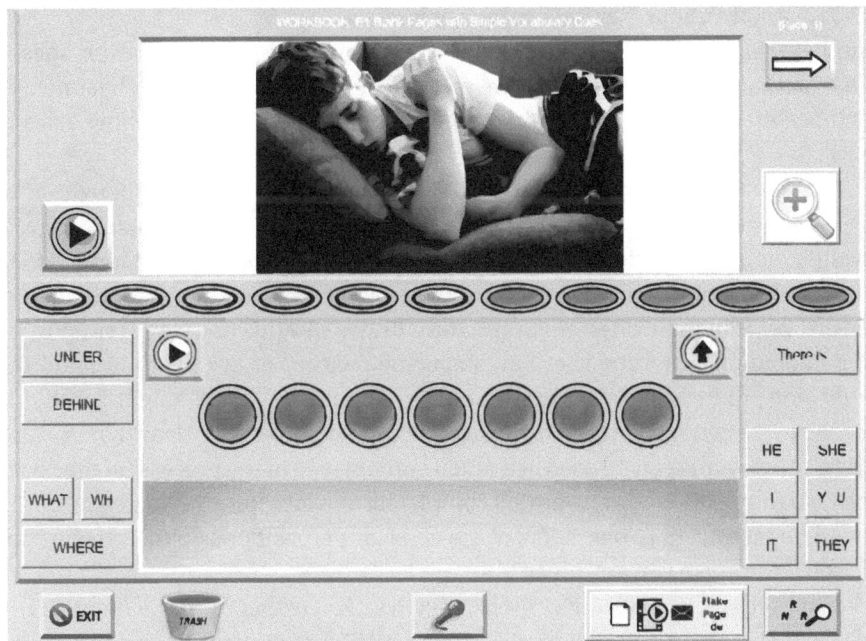

Fig. 9.9: Screen in a personal workbook; Make Video Button on lower right.

Despite these additional features, the core functionality of SentenceShaper is "low tech" as speech technology. It records speech and, through its visual interface, lets users organize their speech recordings into larger structures.

It is clear how this design can provide memory support at the single word level: once the user has retrieved a word, its snippet can simply be replayed. In the Sentence Row, the user's ordering of snippets is saved and does not need to be held in memory; the user can replay the sequence to check its grammatical correctness or search for more words to complete it. Finally, in the Story Row, previous sentences can be replayed in order to keep message-level content activated.

This playback feature also fosters self-monitoring. One impact of the processing limitations hypothesized for aphasia is that users may not have the resources to listen to their own speech after it has been produced (Oomen, Postma & Kolk 2001). This can impact speech not only by preventing error detection, but also because self-monitoring can serve as a kind of self-priming, keeping the words and structures in a sentence activated as the user struggles to put it all together.

9.3.2.2 A note about "lexical bootstrapping"

Another way in which SentenceShaper can help people to create better speech is by facilitating a technique that we will call "lexical bootstrapping": launching sentence creation by starting with a specific word in hand and finding ways to use it.

The default version of SentenceShaper incorporated what we thought of as a lexical survival kit: a set of very general verbs (e.g. "go", "get", "take", "have", "want", etc.), along with a basic set of prepositions. Marshall and Cairns (2005) employed a similar technique, training participants to use a small set of very general verbs in their video retellings. Initially, we saw this as a way of supporting circumlocution when the user had a specific concept or even verb in mind but could not produce it. For example, a user looking for "grab" might be able to use the more general verb "take" instead. However, it became clear that in many cases, these words can be used at a much earlier stage in the process, in the "back end", so to speak. When a user was completely at a loss for what to say, he or she would be instructed to play some of the verbs or prepositions on the side buttons to "see if they give you any ideas".

This technique was often quite effective. For example, participant S11 in Schwartz, Linebarger, Brooks and Bartlett (2007) was attempting to describe her family's celebration of Christmas, but was only able to produce the single word "tree". But when she was instructed to play prepositional side buttons and incorporate them into sentences, she produced the following:

> *Underneath* the tree is a manger. *Above* the manger is a star. In front of the manger, Mary and Joseph are kneeling. *Behind* the tree is a plug. *From* the light *to* the plug, lights are sparkling.

Only the italicized words were provided by SentenceShaper (on the side buttons). All other material was produced spontaneously by the participant.

This technique, of starting with a word and looking for an opportunity to use it in a particular context – of taking it into the "back end" at the interface of language and thought – has not yet been studied systematically, although most clinicians who have worked with SentenceShaper have found it very effective for some but not all users with non-fluent aphasia. It should be noted that it does not feel natural; participant S11 above had to be coaxed to use this technique despite its obvious effectiveness.

One can see why it might help: it serves as a kind of starter for a proposition, thereby (1) cutting down the search space and (2) activating contextually appropriate associates of that item.

9.3.2.3 SentenceShaper's "aided effects": theoretical implications

As discussed above, there is a substantial literature supporting what has been called the performance hypothesis: the view that slow activation and retrieval – as opposed to outright loss of grammatical competence – underlies the fragmented and ungrammatical speech observed in non-fluent aphasia.

This view makes a clear prediction: because SentenceShaper artificially enlarges the user's workspace for language, the program should allow people with non-fluent aphasia to create better speech on it than they can create without this memory support.

This prediction was confirmed in a study (Linebarger et al. 2000) in which six people with agrammatic aphasia learned how to create spoken narratives with SentenceShaper and then practiced using the program for approximately 15 hours. After this, they retold wordless videos (which they had never seen before) with and without SentenceShaper. Importantly, the version of the system used in this study provided no word-finding help at all, just memory support. That is, the vocabulary side buttons and WordFinder were disabled.

The aided narratives (those produced with the program) were longer and more grammatically structured than the unaided versions (those produced spontaneously, without use of SentenceShaper) for five of the six participants. For two of these participants, the contrast between aided and unaided narratives was quite striking.

For example, recall the sample of agrammatic speech above, describing a scene in which a boy enters a fish store while the owner is hitting a fish with a mallet. The boy reaches for the fish and his hand is hit by the mallet. Below are the descriptions of this scene without and with SentenceShaper, by the same participant.

> *Without SentenceShaper:* "Ooh! A fish! Ah, water" and ... uh mmm and attendant, "here", and bumped his head. "Oh boy, oh my hand, my hand, my hand".
> *With SentenceShaper:* The boy and the fishmonger is taking the fish. The boy hit his hand.

Since no word-finding support was provided by SentenceShaper during the elicitation of these descriptions, the increased structure observed in the second description represents the impact of processing support alone.

We will refer to such positive contrasts between aided and unaided speech as "aided effects". Robust aided effects have also been reported in a number of other studies (Linebarger, McCall & Berndt 2002; Linebarger, Schwartz, Kantner & McCall 2002; Bartlett, Fink, Schwartz & Linebarger 2007; Linebarger, Romania, Fink, Bartlett & Schwartz 2008; Albright & Purves 2008). Bartlett et al. (2007)

and Fink, Bartlett, Lowery, Linebarger and Schwartz (2008) have also shown that the program's aided effects appear in measures of the Correct Information Unit (CIU) analysis (Nicholas & Brookshire, 1993) and listener ratings as well as in the measures of the Quantitative Production Analysis (QPA) methodology (Saffran, Berndt & Schwartz 1989). The QPA, widely used in aphasia research, is computed over a transcript from which false starts, repetitions, and non-narrative remarks have been removed, providing a purely structural characterization of the speaker's output in terms of approximately 20 measures.

9.3.2.4 Impact of narrative-based therapy with SentenceShaper

Another effect that has been studied is the impact of SentenceShaper on spontaneous speech. In other words, if people use SentenceShaper for a period, will their spontaneous, unaided speech get better? We will refer to such improvements as "treatment effects". So aided effects are effects *with* versus *without* the program, whereas treatment effects compare speech *before* versus *after* use of the program for a period.

When talking about SentenceShaper as a treatment tool, we are referring primarily to the use of the program for narrative production. There are other treatment tasks for which SentenceShaper may also be effective (e.g. practicing specific structures through traditional picture description drills), but most studies have focused upon the program's more unique ability to facilitate narrative production: creating multi-sentence narratives is difficult or impossible for some individuals without the kind of memory support provided by SentenceShaper. As noted above, narrative production is a highly desirable treatment task, for two reasons: it requires "thinking for speaking" and improved narrative production is in and of itself a functionally relevant treatment goal.

A number of studies (Linebarger et al. 2001; Linebarger, McCall, Virata & Berndt 2007; McCall, Virata, Linebarger & Berndt 2009; Albright & Purves 2008; Hickin, Mehta & Dipper 2015) have reported improvements in unaided narratives – that is, narratives produced without the use of a computer – after a period of using SentenceShaper. In all these treatment studies, the program was used primarily for the construction of multi-sentence narratives, retelling TV shows, movies, or life events. In most cases, participants worked on the program at home and came into the laboratory for training and for weekly observation.

Since these research studies are all small studies with varying protocols and varying outcomes, we cannot make broad claims about the program's efficacy. A representative study is by Linebarger, McCall, Virata and Berndt (2007). This study used a narrative-based SentenceShaper treatment, and participants worked at home after training in the laboratory and came in weekly for observation and testing. Unaided narratives elicited repeatedly at baseline showed no structural or content gains until SentenceShaper treatment commenced. Post-treatment, five of the six participants made significant gains in at least one measure of structure or content and speech rate increased in two participants.

For example, Tab. 9.1 shows the first five utterances produced in unaided narratives (without SentenceShaper) pre and post by participant MR.

A similar improvement was observed in the first phase of a case study by McCall et al. (2009). After a period of narrative-based SentenceShaper treatment, the participant CI's unaided narratives of a wordless picture book showed increased structure and complexity. His mean sentence length, for example, showed a striking increase, from 3.6 to 8.12. Shown in Tab. 9.2 are the first five utterances of his unaided narratives pre and post this phase of treatment.

As indicated above, some people do not show any impact of SentenceShaper use, even an aided effect. Others show aided effects, but these effects do not generalize to unaided narrative production.

Tab. 9.1: First five utterances produced in unaided narratives pre and post by participant MR (Linebarger et al. 2007).

Pre-treatment, without SentenceShaper	Post-treatment, without SentenceShaper
Boy is making a snowman	The kid going to make a stoman [snowman] while the parents are in the house
He rest	The snowman and the kid goes in the house to play with the toys
He went downstairs	He cat screams at the stoman [snowman]
Snowman was light it up	The snowman and the kid goes out to play with the other stoman [snowman]
He brought snowman inside house	He flies with the kid over the neighborhood and flies to the other snowman at lights

Tab. 9.2: First five utterances of participant CI's unaided narratives pre and post first phase of treatment (McCall et al. 2009).

Pre-treatment, without SentenceShaper	Post-treatment, without SentenceShaper
Frog in the bottle	The boy and the frog is having a good time
Frog in the top	The frog is getting out of the jar
Frog in the window	The boy and the frog are sleeping
Frog gone	The boy and the dog are aware the frog is gone
Frog looking at the bottle	The frog in the boot

The nature of the effects also varies across users. While most participants in SentenceShaper studies have been people with non-fluent aphasia whose speech is characterized by fragmentation and ungrammaticality and who show structural gains such as increased sentence length and well-formedness, one participant (SL) in the Linebarger et al. (2007) study entered with a normal proportion of sentences in his connected speech. For this participant, the problem appeared to be largely lexical/semantic in nature. He showed no gains on the QPA structural measures, but instead showed significant change on the content (CIU) measure and the content-related rate measure (CIUs/min), both of which started from a very low baseline.

SL's improvement almost certainly reflects the impact of self-monitoring made possible by SentenceShaper. McCall, Virata, Linebarger and Berndt (2006) presented samples (Tab. 9.3) of the first 2 minutes of SLs unaided video retellings before and after SentenceShaper narrative-based treatment. Notice that the pre-treatment sample contains numerous completely unrelated lexical items: there is nothing in the video about brass candles or bullets or events such as mapping a measured snowstorm.

Tab. 9.3: First 2 minutes of participant SL's unaided video retellings before and after SentenceShaper narrative-based treatment (McCall et al. 2006).

Pre-treatment: 35% of words are CIUs (in bold)

"It brings good things to life **first the snowman** makes a brass candles and two foot **nose and three little** jelly beans **on his** blouse and a green sweater green um green um and **a green hat then** he **put** his nose in the business as far as kid could see **he** mapped a measure measured snowstorm and **goes** by **the woods then he** plays **in the woods for couple of** hours and then he picks up the rainbow and switch **the little boy** on his /ap/ to the rose and then **he comes back to the** bullets and he makes peace with them **he went to** same thing on snowman on snowman"

Post-treatment: 64% of words are CIUs (in bold)

"This is the boy and the snowman story **the boy goes out** and **plays in the snow in the meantime he got on his mind to make a snowman** and **he piles snow in the big round ball** then **he goes in the house** and plays **with the mother and gets the tea and some butter milk biscuits** and **then he goes outside** and plants **a snow head on the body** and then **he goes inside** and plays with the excuse me and **asks his mother if he can have a hat** and a snow bunny **then she says okay** and **he goes out** and **puts the hat on** and **the** snow muffler **to the** snow bunny **then he goes out to the** shop and **gets coal for the snow** bunny's buttons and **then he goes to the** other shack and **gets some for the nose** and then his father **calls him in for supper** and **then he goes to bed then in the morning he wakes up** excuse me"

9.3.2.5 Using SentenceShaper to train specific structures

While most treatment studies with SentenceShaper have focused upon narrative production, the program can also be used for treatments targeting specific structures. In the second part of the McCall et al.'s (2009) study, SentenceShaper was used to train a set of subordinate conjunctions ("before", "after", "because"). The side button cues played these words along with other vocabulary and the clinician began by eliciting sentences with loaded prompts, such as "Why did the woman spill paint on the cat?" The participant used SentenceShaper to construct a response such as "The woman spilled paint on the cat because the boy pulled her". Eventually, the participant was weaned away from these loaded prompts and was simply instructed to create a sentence using "because" or one of the other trained conjunctions. In a sense, the participant was asked to do lexical bootstrapping with the trained item. In many cases, the picture stimulus was not one that had been created for this purpose; for example, the participant was asked to create a sentence with "because" for a picture in which a woman is boiling corn while her family sits at the dinner table.

This second phase of treatment resulted in still further gains in CI's unaided narratives. His mean sentence length, which had increased from 3.6 to 8.12 during the first phase of treatment, increased still further to 11.56 after this second intervention.

Another finding from this second treatment adds support to the performance hypothesis, the view that performance limitations rather than a syntactic deficit underlie the syntactically impoverished and disordered speech observed in nonfluent aphasia. During this treatment, we observed the emergence of personal pronouns in CI's speech. Subordinate clauses frequently refer to entities that are also arguments of the main clause; for example, in CI's sentence, "The boy is cutting his grapes before he eats them", there are three instances of pronominal reference ("the boy" serves as antecedent of both "his" and "he", and "the grapes" is the antecedent of "them"). Not only did the incidence of pronoun use increase markedly following treatment, but CI never violated grammatical rules on intra-sentential pronominal anaphora; for example, he never created a sentence like "*He is cutting his grapes before the boy eats them", where *he* and *the boy* are intended to refer to the same person. This is significant because CI was not instructed in the principles of pronominal reference during this study.

SentenceShaper was subsequently modified to incorporate workbooks targeting "because". These workbooks were incorporated into the successful single-participant treatment intervention reported in Hickin, Dipper, and Mehta (2015).

9.3.3 Interleaving drill with narrative production: TS and SentenceShaper together

Another study involving both narrative production and exercises targeting a particular structure is reported in Linebarger et al. (2001). In this study, both the "TS" program – which incorporated speech recognition and natural language understanding to drill specific prepositional structures – and SentenceShaper were used. In two case studies reported in the paper, modules of TS training were interleaved with use of SentenceShaper. The performance of participant JT illustrates with particular clarity the potential roles of drilling and narrative production.

JT's therapy consisted of a series of modules (approximately 15 hours, largely at home) in which he used either the TS or the SentenceShaper. In the first module, called "CS (Communication System)" training,[4] he created free narratives on SentenceShaper. This was followed by the "Locative Assertions" module, in which he simple sentences like "The bird is behind the cup", using the TS. This was followed by a period of SentenceShaper use (termed the "CS/Prepositions" module) in which he constructed free narratives but was instructed to use prepositions as much as possible in his narratives. The prepositions were available on the side buttons.

Over the course of the entire experiment, JT showed striking improvements in structural measures of production in his unaided video narratives. For example, median length of utterance increased from 2 to 6, and mean sentence length from 3.7 to 7.1.

The video narratives collected at each point in training allowed us to track the effect of each module on JT's narrative production. The first period of SentenceShaper use (the "CS Training" module) resulted in marked structural gains in unaided narratives. JT's family reported that he began speaking more at home following this module, and indeed, these gains were maintained and consolidated during a 3-month absence. Following the Locative Assertions module of the TS, JT actually declined in several of these measures, but showed improved production of locative picture descriptions. Despite his improved production of prepositions in these single-picture description tasks JT still used prepositions very rarely in the more unconstrained task of video retelling after this module. The 150-word sample used for assessment contained no prepositions at all following Locative Assertions training. In the full transcript of 522 narrative words produced following Locative Assertions training, there were only two preposi-

---

4 Recall that SentenceShaper was referred to as "CS" (communication system) in publications prior to 2006.

tions. But following the CS/Prepositions module, in which he was instructed to use prepositions in the narratives he created at home with SentenceShaper, preposition use increased in the unaided narratives elicited after this module. The number of prepositions in his unaided narratives increased from 0 to 12 in the 150-word composite and from 2 to 39 in the combined narrative words of both videos.

This pattern of improvement illustrates the benefits of combining drilling, to activate words and structures, and free narrative creation, to use them in thinking for speaking. The focused drilling provided by the TS was necessary to activate prepositional structures, but narrative creation on SentenceShaper was required to bring them into JT's open-ended narratives. The processing support provided by SentenceShaper, along with the vocabulary cues provided in this module, made this exercise possible.

The second participant in this study, JW, showed a less clear-cut pattern of preposition acquisition, probably because he started with greater mastery of prepositions. His preposition use increased following the first module of SentenceShaper use, prior to the TS preposition module. However, JW made gains in narrative measures (e.g. his MLU increased from 4 pre to 6.5 post, and mean sentence length increased from 6.3 to 8).

9.3.4 SentenceShaper research: some bottom lines

- SentenceShaper's aided effects – that is, the superiority of speech produced with the program to the same user's spontaneous speech – have been reported for a variety of measures (QPA, CIU, informativeness ratings).
- The finding that speech produced on SentenceShaper – with no word-finding support provided by the program or by the experimentor – is superior to the same speakers' spontaneous speech provides striking support for the "processing limitations" account of agrammatic/non-fluent sentence production in aphasia. Simply providing memory support can increase the length, complexity, well-formedness, and informativeness of speech in agrammatic aphasia.
- Because SentenceShaper makes it possible for people with non-fluent aphasia to create multi-sentence narratives, treatment interventions with the program have exploited this capability and have typically focused upon aided narrative production. A set of small studies has demonstrated treatment effects, sometimes marked, in some but not all speakers. In contrast, most speakers with non-fluent aphasia show aided effects, especially with support by a clinician or helper.

9.3.5 Future directions: using SentenceShaper to enhance life participation

SentenceShaper's core functionality helps people with non-fluent aphasia to create more complex and well-formed sentences and messages than they are able to produce without the aid. This makes it possible to demonstrate to others that they are still able to think and formulate complicated ideas, that is, to express their identity more fully. In addition, features such as the creation of videos combining users' personal pictures with their recorded speech and the ability to e-mail these from within the program are potentially valuable in terms of enhancing users' social connectedness and life participation.

These features, while valuable, do not draw upon any additional kinds of speech technology. As a speech application, SentenceShaper remains relatively low tech: it simply records the user's speech. However, there are ways in which SentenceShaper could in fact be extended to incorporate or support other kinds of speech technology in order to enhance life participation.

As noted above, SentenceShaper records users' utterances but does not analyze them. For example, it does not (in contrast to our screenshots) display the text of each snippet that the user records. Why not? It is unlikely that automatic speech recognition (ASR) technology is currently accurate enough to recognize the utterances of people with ungrammatical, often distorted, speech, in a situation where there is (in contrast to the TS and speech-enabled therapy applications in which the target is known) no constraint on the expected topic. This is especially true at the level of snippets, which may contain no more than a single word.

As a result, it could easily disrupt the process of sentence construction to involve the user in recording speech, playing it back, integrating it into a sentence with other snippets, and simultaneously "vetting" the text produced by the speech recognizer. However, if a user is specifically motivated to produce text, then performing speech recognition within SentenceShaper might be quite helpful. It is an optional feature that we will explore in future versions of the program.

And the program already has the potential to support speech recognition for people with aphasia. One possibility is for users to create recorded utterances with SentenceShaper, and then submit these recordings to a speech recognizer. Dahl, Linebarger and Berndt (2008) explored the idea of using SentenceShaper as an interface to speech recognition in this way. We compared the recognition of spoken narratives recorded (under acoustically identical conditions) with and without SentenceShaper. For three of the four participants, recognition was more accurate for the aided narratives.

Another way for the program to support speech recognition is by serving as a platform for assembling and practicing utterances before submitting them directly to the speech recognizer. That is, the user would create a sentence on SentenceShaper, but would then repeat it "live" into the microphone to submit it directly to the speech recognizer. This can be accomplished by running a program like wordQ+speakQ (2015) simultaneously with SentenceShaper; the text of the recognizer appears within the optional text area on the SentenceShaper screen.

Another speech technology that would seem to have a natural synergy with SentenceShaper is voice-based Internet communication activities such as skyping and video conferencing. Users could prepare more complex utterances such as anecdotes or questions ahead of a call, then play them into the call as needed, intermingling them with live speech. We plan to explore this in future versions of SentenceShaper. More generally, see Linebarger, Romania et al. (2008) for a fuller discussion of the potential, and the challenges, of incorporating pre-recorded speech into real-time communications.

9.4 Survey of speech technology for sentence production

In the previous sections, we have provided a detailed account of the development and deployment of two speech technology programs, the "TS" and SentenceShaper. We turn now to a broader look at the kinds of speech applications that have been developed – or can be used – to help people with aphasic sentence production disorders. Note that our focus is on speech at the sentence level and beyond, since previous chapters have addressed software targeting single word retrieval. Also, because technology evolves so rapidly, we recommend that you consult resources like the Aphasia Software Finder website (2015) to stay abreast of new software.

As noted earlier, there are three major ways in which speech technology can support language production in aphasia: (1) by analyzing the user's speech (turning it into text and possibly determining its intended meaning); (2) by recording and playing back the user's speech; and (3) by transmitting the user's speech to others.

9.4.1 Software that analyzes the user's speech

Technology that analyzes the user's speech, by turning it into text and possibly determining its intended meaning, can serve the following goals:
–   To give feedback about correctness and completeness;
–   To enable the user to engage in complex tasks;

- To create a text transcript;
- To analyze speech patterns for diagnostic purposes.

These goals are discussed separately below.

9.4.1.1 Goal: To give feedback about correctness and completeness

Analyzing the user's spoken input can allow us to tell her whether or not her utterance is correct or complete and perhaps even to point out errors and omissions. The first program we discussed above, the TS, used speech recognition and natural language understanding for this purpose. The TS has not been commercially released, and at this time, we are not aware of any commercially available aphasia software that analyzes the grammatical structure of user's sentences so thoroughly and provides such detailed feedback.

However, it is quite possible that "less is more" and that the full grammatical analysis of the user's entire utterance performed by the TS was overkill. It may be that less ambitious uses of speech recognition might be just as good, or even better. In the category of "less ambitious" uses of ASR, we include word spotting (just looking for specific words or phrases in the user's input) or simply matching the user's input to an expected utterance. Recall that the TS obtained a text string from the speech recognizer (e.g. "the clown pushes the dancer into the pool") and then submitted this string to grammatical and semantic analysis. Feedback was based upon the presence of a correct verb and/or preposition and also the presence of the correct arguments. In contrast, the "less ambitious" technique of word spotting might just look for certain words in the utterance (the verb, noun, and prepositions) and utterance matching would just compare the recognizer's transcript with an expected utterance (or possibly multiple utterances). These techniques were not used in the TS because listing all the possible utterances for a given picture, taking into consideration the possibility of users' employing synonyms and making morphological/function word errors, would have led to a combinatorial explosion of possible sentences. More importantly, it would not have allowed the program to give feedback about errors and omissions.

At the sentence level, few commercially available programs use speech recognition in applications targeting sentence production. However, Parrot Software (2015) offers a suite of sentence production programs that draw on speech recognition. The Parrot speech-enabled programs incorporate what we described above as "less ambitious" uses of speech technology (word spotting, utterance matching) than those employed by the TS. We will examine a few of these programs briefly here because they demonstrate some benefits of this approach, and also illustrate the potential variety of tasks and feedback that speech-enabled applications for sentence production can provide.

Parrot offers different speech recognition options, including the Google speech recognizer (built into the Chrome browser), which performed very well in our testing. Some speech recognition issues arise with homophones, punctuation marks, and user dysfluencies, but for people who can produce the target sentence relatively fluently, the speech recognition can be quite accurate.

Utterance Matching: Parrot's *Mastering Personal Information* exemplifies a simple but very flexible utterance matching paradigm. The clinician or helper types in a set of prompt/response pairs, e.g. a prompt "What is your name?" and a required response "My name is Margaret". When the user runs the program, the prompt is played aloud by text-to-speech (TTS) and the user must say (without seeing the text) the listed response, verbatim. Feedback is provided about correctness; the response must match the expected response perfectly. The program is extremely flexible; it could be used for therapy exercises training specific structures (for example, a prompt "Ask me if I like coffee" could be paired with a required response "Do you like coffee?") or for memorizing scripts. Given the high accuracy of the speech recognition (especially with Google Chrome), this simple program exemplifies a very straightforward and flexible speech application.

A program under development by other developers, BangaSpeak (Messamer, Ramsberger & Atkins in press) resembles *Mastering Personal Information* in its basic structure, but is augmented with several important features such as the ability to display images, add hints, and easily create new treatment materials. Each treatment item consists of a picture and an expected response, along with optional hints. Like the Parrot program, BangaSpeak incorporates exact utterance matching, although it examines the top five hypotheses on the N-best list, providing more flexibility.

Word Spotting: Several other programs by Parrot request full sentences but rely on word spotting rather than full syntactic analysis to provide feedback. *Say a Sentence* displays a picture of an object and instructs the user to say a sentence that contains the word pictured in the image AND starts with a particular word (for example, "I"). Thus, if the pictured image is a car, the user may be instructed to create a sentence beginning with "I" and containing "car" (for example, "I have a car" or "I want a car"). Speech recognition is only used to determine the presence of those two words, and there is no linguistic analysis of the user's speech. Similarly, *Saying Present Progressive Verbs* displays a video of a verb action and asks the user to produce a sentence with the verb. However, it only checks for the verb in giving feedback. In both of these programs, it seems possible that the task promotes thinking for speaking (forcing the user to imagine, and then verbalize, a proposition incorporating certain elements). The use of simple word spotting rather than full-blown syntactic analysis actually makes this possible, because more detailed feedback about correctness would require that the program present a picture, or in some way constrain the range of likely responses. That is, the open-ended nature of the task has costs (no feedback about the appropriateness or grammaticality of the user's full sentence) but also benefits (potentially valuable, VNeST-like practice in activating appropriate verbs and arguments).

Regarding feedback, the evidence for relatively preserved grammatical knowledge in agrammatism raises the question of whether explicit feedback about correctness is necessary. Perhaps more of a concern is that, as noted above, impaired self-monitoring may limit the effect of corrections because speakers may not be clear about what exactly they said, especially if it was more than a word or two.

Nonetheless, given the need for treatment intensity, motivation is extremely important, and successful speech recognition makes it possible to provide potentially motivating feedback about correctness. "Getting it right" may be especially important to overcome the tedium of drilling and other repetitive tasks.

Of course, feedback about correctness is not the only way to engage the user. Speech technology can support a wide range of human-computer interactions, which may prove motivating and which may also support language practice in a more naturalistic way.

9.4.1.2 Goal: To enable the user to engage in complex tasks

Consider, for example, tasks in which the user is rewarded by accomplishing some kind of goal. In barrier games, users have to communicate information to another person. Maher et al. (2006) (Maher et al. 2006) trained participants to create sentences such as "Bill, do you have the three red books?" in a dual card task. One can imagine that the feedback of actually gaining a card by describing it correctly to a virtual listener who does not know what is on the card might be more motivating, and even more therapeutic (by increasing awareness of what the listener needs to know) than the feedback provided by programs like the TS, which simply tell the user whether their sentence correctly describes a picture. Similarly, even in a highly pre-scripted interaction, such as a dialog with a store clerk in which the user is shown a picture of items to ask for, actually receiving the item on the screen might have considerable impact.

Parrot's *Talk Your Way Through a Maze* exemplifies this kind of feedback, in a very primitive way. The program allows users to navigate their way through a maze by speaking directions (limited to, unfortunately, "up", "down", "left", "right"). One could imagine that navigating more complex environments such as a virtual reality world could prove highly motivating; for example, if two avatars need to arrange a meeting place in a virtual reality world.

Another potential use of speech technology is open-ended dialog practice with a computerized partner, which might provide not only language practice but also train the speaker to pay more attention to the needs of the listener. Technology for natural language generation would obviously need to be incorporated in most dialog applications. Virtual reality environments offer an ideal venue for interactive dialog applications.

Speech-enabled programs designed for the general public can provide feedback that comes in the form of accomplishing some functional task, rather than simply being informed of the correctness of one's utterance. Personal assistant programs such as Siri (2009), and speech-enabled search engines such as Google Voice Search, are in increasingly wide use among people with aphasia. In addition to their practical usefulness, these programs represent a kind of "barrier game" in the sense that (in contrast to, e.g. a picture description task) the computer does not know what the user is trying to say.

9.4.1.3 Goal: To create a text transcript

Another reason to analyze the user's speech is to create a text transcript. Speech recognition systems for dictation (e.g. Dragon Naturally Speaking 2015, wordQ+speakQ and Write:OutLoud® 2015) have been used successfully with people with relatively mild aphasia (Bruce, Emundson & Coleman 2003; Hickin et al. 2015). In addition to providing access to text for those who have impaired reading and writing, dictation systems also provide memory support, since the user has access to previous utterances, which can be replayed via TTS. In addition, dictation software usually incorporates error correction and word prediction. Dictation software can therefore serve both assistive and therapeutic purposes. Hickin et al. employed both Dragon NaturallySpeaking Premium and SentenceShaper in a treatment program for a woman with mild non-fluent aphasia, and reported significant improvements in (unaided) narrative production.

The challenges of speech recognition for people with aphasia include the following:
- Intelligibility issues resulting from dysarthria and apraxia can obviously hinder recognition.
- Syntactic fragmentation in users' speech is a problem, since speech recognition typically relies upon models that incorporate grammatical information.
- Impaired executive function or other cognitive impairments may make it harder for the user to operate a speech recognizer: turning it on and off, speaking as clearly as possible without interjections ("I know it but I can't say it"), and correcting recognition errors.

Some of these problems may be eased with additional support, whether the processing support provided by SentenceShaper (described above) or simply more user-friendly interfaces for people with language impairments.

9.4.1.4 Goal: To analyze speech patterns for diagnostic purposes

Another reason to analyze spoken utterances is to be able to determine the speaker's linguistic and/or cognitive abilities. This would help in diagnosis and also in tracking the impact of different treatment interventions. It is very hard to compare treatments unless they all measure the same functionally relevant aspects of language.

Speech technology that recognizes users' speech has considerable potential in this regard, and there is a growing body of work on the use of automated analysis of narratives to diagnose different aphasic and cognitive impairments (Coulston, Klabbers, De Villiers & Hosom 2007; Lehr, Prud'hommeaux, Shafran & Roark 2012; Fraser, Rudzicz, Graham & Rochon 2013; Fraser et al. 2014).

Above, we have examined several purposes for automated analysis of aphasic speech: to provide feedback about correctness; to make it possible for the user to practice language by engaging in a variety of interactions with the computer; to create a text transcript of the user's speech, whether to enhance social connectedness or for language therapy; or, finally, to help diagnose different impairments and track the user's language skills during treatment interventions.

9.4.2 Software that records and plays back the user's speech

We turn now to a second form of speech technology: software that records and plays back the user's speech.

How can this functionality support language production in aphasia?
- It may, depending upon the design of the program, allow users to edit their speech, correcting and expanding their utterances.
- It can let users compare their utterances to a model.
- It can enhance communication by allowing users to share their recorded speech with others.

9.4.2.1 Goal: To allow users to edit their speech

SentenceShaper, already discussed above, is an example of this kind of speech technology. It records but does not analyze the user's speech. By allowing users to replay and evaluate their own utterances, it provides memory support (access to previously uttered words, phrases, or sentences) and facilitates self-monitoring. It is, in a sense, a word processor for speech.

9.4.2.2 Goal: To let users compare their speech to a model

Recording users' speech also allows them to determine whether or not their utterances are correct. For example, Bungalow Software's Sights 'n Sounds 2 (2015) allows users to play back their recorded version of a sentence and compare it to the program's spoken model. Similarly, SentenceShaper includes built-in workbooks that target specific structures with single-picture description tasks, and in these workbooks, users can compare their utterances to a pre-recorded model.

This process of checking the correctness of one's utterances oneself – rather than being informed of their correctness by the software – offers the potential benefit of encouraging the user to self-monitor. However, as noted above, this is almost certainly less entertaining – and hence less motivating – than receiving feedback from the program itself. We are not aware of any studies that directly compare these two kinds of feedback.

9.4.2.3 Goal: To enhance communication

Although software that merely records speech cannot provide feedback about correctness, it can provide a different kind of motivation: sharing one's recorded speech with others. This in itself may motivate the user to spend more time creating speech, which can engender treatment effects.

The current version of SentenceShaper (2015) incorporates tools to create videos that combine the user's aided speech and any personal photos and allows the user to e-mail these videos from within the program. Videos or other presentations created on SentenceShaper (2015) have also been used for speeches, played on handheld devices Linebarger et al. (2008) and posted on Vimeo and Facebook. Data are sparse on the extent to which these features increase motivation to use SentenceShaper, although a qualitative study (True, Bartlett, Fink, Linebarger & Schwartz 2010) reported largely positive responses from aphasic users.

There are a variety of other commercial programs that record speech and combine it with pictures and text. For example, *Pictello* by AssistiveWare® (Pictello 2015) is especially easy to use and allows the user to combine recorded speech with pictures, offering users a variety of methods to share their creations. Unlike SentenceShaper, it can incorporate TTS for playback. However, it lacks SentenceShaper's processing support for message creation and its direct support for e-mailing productions.

More generally, the sound recorders available for any smartphone can be used to record speech, although their interfaces are rarely user-friendly for people with aphasia, hemiplegia, and/or reading impairments.

Software that records the user's speech can also be used as an AAC aid to support real-time communications. That is, the person with aphasia can pre-record utterances and then play her recordings to others or instead can use these recordings to self-cue live speech. Linebarger et al. (2008) describe a pilot study of the use of pre-recorded SentenceShaper for self-cued communication assistance.

9.4.3 Software that transmits the user's speech

Finally, as noted above, a third operation that speech technology can perform on the user's speech is to transmit it to others.

This category includes general purpose technology like Skype, Facetime, Webex, and so forth, which can play an important role in delivering therapy over the Internet and facilitating communication for people with aphasia, who typically have impaired reading and writing. Unfortunately, however, they are not always easy for people with aphasia to navigate without some kind of support from a clinician or helper.

Virtual reality environments for people with aphasia may soon provide a powerful venue for the transmission of users' speech. Typically, these environments offer the opportunity to explore visually interesting landscapes and rehearse functionally relevant interactions such as ordering in a restaurant. Users can communicate with others by speaking into a microphone. Although many of these environments may be dauntingly complex for people who are also dealing with a language impairment, more aphasia-friendly virtual environments are being developed. For example, the EVA Project (2015; Wilson et al. 2015) is developing an aphasia-friendly world named Eva Park, using Open Simulator, an open-source platform for creating multiuser, three-dimensional virtual environments.

Again, we note that all these different speech technologies can be synergistic. For example, the speech transmitted in Skype calls or virtual reality applications might be prepared ahead of time by the user, using other technology (e.g. pre-recording on software such as SentenceShaper or creating with a dictation program such as speakQ+thoughtQ, Dragon, or Write:OutLoud). The user could then use this prepared speech to self-cue live speech or, in the case of text, transmit it as a text message within the call or virtual reality application.

9.4.4 Helpful software not covered in this chapter

Finally, we mention some worthwhile software that falls on the periphery of the scope we have defined for this chapter.

9.4.4.1 Iconic communication aids

There are a rich variety of devices and programs that can help people with aphasia to communicate. AAC devices that play pre-stored utterances via synthesized or recorded speech (e.g. DynaVox 2015, Lingraphica® 2009, TouchSpeak™ 2015, Proloquo2Go 2015) can be used to replace speech or to cue live speech. They are not treated in this chapter because they do not take the user's speech as input.

9.4.4.2 Software for script training

For the same reason, we have not discussed two valuable programs that are designed to help users produce scripts, whether for practice or for use in conversation. AphasiaScripts™ is a program to help people with aphasia practice specific scripts. It incorporates "virtual therapists", animated agents who speak the scripts, modeling appropriate movements of the speech articulators. Video Assisted Speech Technology (VAST 2015) is a service that creates video recordings of a clinician speaking sentences or scripts provided by the user. The videos provide lip cues and other support for fluent speech to support functional communication and/or language therapy. Scripts can also be created and practiced using speech technology discussed above (e.g. speakQ+wordQ, SentenceShaper).

9.4.4.3 Speech recognition to support comprehension

Although our focus here is on technology to support language production, ASR can also play a role for individuals with language comprehension impairments. An ingenious use of speech recognition is described by Ramsberger and Messamer (2014), who deployed a smartphone speech recognition app for use by *conversational partners* of an individual with Wernicke's aphasia. The client's auditory comprehension was impaired, in contrast to relatively preserved understanding of written text. Conversational partners spoke into the phone and then showed the client the text of their utterances. This, in effect, captioned the non-aphasic person's speech, making it easier for the client to understand. The authors note that this process also helped to retrain the habit of conversational turn-taking.

9.4.4.4 Software to track speech activity

Finally, CommFit (Brandenburg, Worrall, Copland, Power & Rodriguez 2015), an app under investigation, is a "talkometer", recording the amount of time that the user speaks out loud on a given day. It falls outside the scope of this chapter because it does not record, analyze, or transmit the user's speech, but simply registers that speech has occurred. However, this information could be potentially quite valuable in tracking progress of treatment interventions as well as in motivating users with aphasia to practice their speech.

9.5 Summary

We have examined three different ways in which computers can act upon the user's spoken input to support communication and to aid in the treatment of aphasic sentence production disorders. The most ambitious goal is to analyze this spoken input: to turn it into text with speech recognition and even to extract elements of meaning relevant to a given task with natural language understanding. We have also observed that the lower-tech operation of simply recording the user's speech can provide crucial processing support for spoken language. Finally, technologies that support the transmission of speech – especially when paired with aphasia-friendly interfaces – are becoming increasingly important in the management of aphasia, through online therapy and Internet-based social activities such as virtual reality worlds.

We have emphasized the synergism of these technologies. For example, software that helps users to construct better sentences (e.g. dictation software or SentenceShaper) can be used for offline message creation. These messages can then be employed for language practice, transmitted to others over the Internet, or used to self-cue live speech, potentially in an Internet-based setting such as a Skype call or a virtual reality world. There is also a synergy between social and therapeutic efforts: activities that foster social connectedness also increase the intensity of language practice.

In the discussion above, we have not explicitly addressed the role of clinicians and other helpers in the use of this technology. Clearly, many people with aphasia require support, and even clinicians are increasingly turning to technology consultants (see, e.g. Ramsberger & Messamer 2014) to help identify and deploy appropriate software. In many cases, however, working together on technology can offer potentially rewarding kinds of social interaction, whether in the home, the clinic, online treatment programs, or aphasia centers. It also is important to stress the value of engaging in participatory design with potential end users. As speech technology continues to mature and to be incorporated into other emerging technologies, it is hard not to be optimistic about its potential to enhance both language and social connectedness in people with aphasia.

References

Albright, E. & Purves, B. (2008). Exploring SentenceShaper: Treatment and augmentative possibilities. *Aphasiology, 22*, 741–752.

Aphasia Software Finder. (2015). Retrieved from http://www.speech-therapy.org.uk/aphasia-software-finder

AphasiaScripts™. (2015). Rehabilitation Institute of Chicago. Retrieved March 18, 2015, from http://ricaphasiascripts.contentshelf.com/welcome

Bartlett, M. R., Fink, R. B., Schwartz, M. F. & Linebarger, M. C. (2007). Informativeness ratings of messages created on an AAC processing prosthesis. *Aphasiology, 21*, 475–498.

Berndt, R. S. & Mitchum, C. C. (1995). Cognitive neuropsychological approaches to the treatment of language disorders. *Neuropsychological Rehabilitation, 5*, 1–6.

Blackwell, A. & Bates, E. (1995). Inducing agrammatic profiles in normals: Evidence for the selective vulnerability of morphology under cognitive resource limitation. *Journal of Cognitive Neuroscience, 7*, 228–257.

Brandenburg, C., Worrall, L., Copland, D., Power, E. & Rodriguez, A. D. (2015). The development and accuracy testing of CommFit™, an iPhone application for individuals with aphasia. *Aphasiology.* DOI: 10.1080/02687038.2015.1028329.

Breitenstein, C., Kamping, S., Jansen, A., Schomacher, M. & Knecht, S. (2004). Word learning can be achieved without feedback: Implications for aphasia therapy. *Restorative Neurology and Neuroscience, 22*, 445–458.

Bruce, C., Emundson, A. & Coleman, M. (2003). Writing with voice: An investigation of the use of a voice recognition system as a writing aid for a man with aphasia. *International Journal of Language & Communication Disorders, 38*, 131–148.

Byng, S. (1988). Sentence processing deficits: Theory and therapy. *Cognitive Neuropsychology, 5*, 629–676.

Byng, S., Nickels, L. & Black, M. (1994). Replicating therapy for mapping deficits in agrammatism: Remapping the deficit. *Aphasiology, 8*, 315–341.

Caplan, D. & Waters, G. S. (1995). Aphasic disorders of syntactic comprehension and working memory capacity. *Cognitive Neuropsychology, 12*, 637–649.

Cherney, L. R., Halper, A. S., Holland, A. L. & Cole, R. (2008). Computerized script training for aphasia: Preliminary results. *American Journal of Speech-Language Pathology, 17*, 19–34.

Coulston, R., Klabbers, E., De Villiers, J. & Hosom, J. P. (2007). Application of speech technology in a home based assessment kiosk for early detection of Alzheimer's disease. *Interspeech*, 2573–2676.

Dahl, D. A., Linebarger, M. C. & Berndt, R. S. (2008). Improving automatic recognition of aphasic speech through the use of a processing prosthesis. *Technology and Disability, 20*, 283–294.

Dipper, L. T., Black, M. & Bryan, K. L. (2005). Thinking for speaking and thinking for listening: The interaction of thought and language in typical and non-fluent comprehension and production. *Language and Cognitive Processes, 20*, 417–441.

Doyle, P. J., Tsironas, D., Goda, A. & Kalinyak, M. (1996). The relationship between objective measures and listeners' judgments of the communicative informativeness of the connected discourse of adults with aphasia. *American Journal of Speech Language Pathology, 5,* 53–60.

Dragon Naturally Speaking. (2015). Retrieved from http://www.nuance.com/dragon/

DynaVox. (2015). Retrieved from http://www.dynavoxtech.com/

Elaine Wolpe Speech. (2015). Retrieved from http://sentenceshaper.com/2012/02/13/a-speech-to-remember/

Emonds, L. A., Nadeau, S. E. & Kiran, S. (2009). Effect of verb network strengthening treatment (VNeST) on lexical retrieval of content words in sentences in persons with aphasia. *Aphasiology, 23,* 402–424.

Fink, R. B., Bartlett, M. R., Lowery, J. S., Linebarger, M. C. & Schwartz, M. F. (2008). Aphasic speech with and without SentenceShaper: Two methods for assessing informativeness. *Aphasiology, 22,* 679–690.

Fraser, K., Rudzicz, F., Graham, N. & Rochon, E. (2013). Automatic speech recognition in the diagnosis of primary progressive aphasia. *Proceedings of the Fourth Workshop on Speech and Language Processing for Assistive Technologies* (pp. 47–54).

Fraser, K. C., Meltzer, J. A., Graham, N. L., Leonard, C., Hirst, G., Black, S. E. & Rochon, E. (2014). Automated classification of primary progressive aphasia subtypes from narrative speech transcripts.*Cortex, 55,* 43–60.

Frattali, C., Thompson, C., Holland, A., Wohl, C. B. & Ferketic, M. (1995). *Functional assessment of communication skills for adults.* Rockville, MD: American Speech-Language-Hearing Association.

Friederici, A. (1982). Syntactic and semantic processes in aphasic deficits: The availability of prepositions. *Brain and Language, 15,* 249–258.

Hartsuiker, R. J. & Kolk, H. H. J. (1998). Syntactic facilitation in agrammatic sentence production. *Brain and Language, 62,* 221–254.

Helm-Estabrooks, N. A. (1981). *Helm elicited language program for syntax stimulation.* Austin, TX: Exceptional Resources.

Hickin, J., Mehta, B. & Dipper, L. (2015). To the sentence and beyond: A single case therapy report for mild aphasia. *Aphasiology,* 1–24.

Jacobs, B. J. (2001). Social validity of changes in informativeness and efficiency of aphasic discourse following linguistic specific treatment. *Brain and Language, 78,* 115–127.

Kempler, D. & Goral, M. (2011). A comparison of drill- and communication-based treatment for aphasia. *Aphasiology, 25,* 1327–1346.

Kolk, H. H. J. (1995). A time-based approach to agrammatic comprehension. *Brain and Language, 50,* 282–303.

Kolk, H. H. J. &, Heeschen, C. (1992). Agrammatism, paragrammatism, and the management of language. *Language and Cognitive Processes, 7,* 82–129.

Lehr, M., Prud'hommeaux, E., Shafran, I. & Roark, B. (2012). Fully automated neuropsychological assessment for detecting mild cognitive impairment. *Interspeech,* 1039–1042.

Lesser, R. (1989). *Some issues in the neuropsychological rehabilitation of anomia.* Hillsdale, NJ: Lawrence Erlbaum.

Levelt, W. J. M. (1989). *Speaking.* Cambridge, MA: MIT Press.

Linebarger, M. C. & Romania, J. F. (inventors) (2000). Unisys Corporation (assignee). System for synthesizing spoken messages. US Patent 6068485.

Linebarger, M. C. & Romania, J. F. (inventors) (2007). *Aphasia therapy system.* US Patent 7203649.

Linebarger, M., McCall, D. & Berndt, R. S. (2002). Retraining narrative production: Impact of processing support. *Brain and Language, 83,* 172–175.

Linebarger, M. C., McCall, D., Galbraith, C., & Fink, R. B. (2015). Empowering Fathers to be Fathers with Voice Email. Poster presented at AphasiaAccess Leadership Summit, March 2015, Boston, MA. (Accessed 2015, at http://sentenceshaper.com/AphasiaAccess2015/)

Linebarger, M. C., McCall, D., Virata, T. & Berndt, R. S. (2007). Widening the temporal window: Processing support in the treatment of aphasic language production. *Brain and Language, 100*, 53–68.

Linebarger, M. C., Romania, J. R., Fink, R. B., Bartlett, M. & Schwartz, M. F. (2008). Building on residual speech: A portable processing prosthesis for aphasia. *Journal of Rehabilitation Research and Development, 45*, 1401–1414.

Linebarger, M. C., Schwartz, M., Kantner, T. R. & McCall, D. (2002). Promoting access to the Internet in aphasia [abstract]. *Brain and Language, 83*, 169–172.

Linebarger, M. C., Schwartz, M. F. & Kohn, S. E. (2001). Computer-based training of language production: An exploratory study. *Neuropsychological Rehabilitation, 11*, 57–96.

Linebarger, M. C., Schwartz, M. F. & Saffran, E. M. (1983). Sensitivity to grammatical structure in so-called agrammatic aphasics. *Cognition, 13*, 361–392.

Linebarger, M. C., Schwartz, M. F., Romania, J. F., Kohn, S. E. & Stephens, D. L. (2000). Grammatical encoding in aphasia: Evidence from a "processing prosthesis". *Brain and Language, 75*, 416–427.

Lingraphica. (2009). http://www.aphasia.com

Maher, L. M., Kendall, D., Swearengin, J. A., Rodriguez, A., Leon, S. A., Pingel, K., Holland, A., Gonzalez Rothi, L. J., Gonzalez Rothi, L. J. (2006). A pilot study of use-dependent learning in the context of constraint induced language therapy. *Journal of the International Neuropsychological Society, 12*, 843–852.

Marshall, J. & Cairns, D. (2005). Therapy for sentence processing problems in aphasia: Working on thinking for speaking. *Aphasiology, 19*, 1009–1020.

Marshall, J., Pring, T. & Chiat, S. (1998). Verb retrieval and sentence production in aphasia. *Brain and Language, 63*, 159–183.

McCall, D., Virata, T., Linebarger, M. & Berndt, R. S. (2009). Integrating technology and targeted treatment to improve narrative production in aphasia: A case study. *Aphasiology, 23*, 438–461.

McCall, D., Virata, T., Linebarger, M. C. & Berndt, R. S. (2006). Retraining narrative production in patients with aphasia. In *Maryland Speech and Hearing Association Annual Convention*, Frederick, MA.

Messamer, P., Ramsberger, G. & Atkins, A. (submitted). Designing apps for clients and SLP users: BangaSpeak – an app example for aphasia.

Mitchum, C. C. & Berndt, R. S. (1994). *Verb retrieval and sentence construction: Effects of targeted intervention*. Hove, UK: Lawrence Erlbaum Associates.

Miyake, A., Carpenter, P. & Just, M. A. (1994). A capacity approach to syntactic comprehension disorders: Making normal adults perform like aphasic patients. *Cognitive Neuropsychology, 11*, 671–717.

Nicholas, L. E. & Brookshire R. H. (1993). A system for quantifying the informativeness and efficiency of the connected speech of adults with aphasia. *Journal of Speech and Hearing Research, 36*, 338–350.

Oomen, C. C. E., Postma, A. & Kolk, H. H. J. (2001). Prearticulatory and postarticulatory self-monitoring in Broca's aphasia. *Cortex, 37*, 627–641.

OpenSimulator. http://opensimulator.org/

Parrot. (2015). http://www.parrotsoftware.com

Peach, R. & Wong, P. (2004). Integrating the message level into treatment for agrammatism using story retelling. *Aphasiology, 18*, 429–441.

Pictello. (2015). Retrieved from http://www.assistiveware.com/product/pictello

Proloquo2Go. (2015). Retrieved from http://www.assistiveware.com/product/proloquo2go

Ramsberger, G. & Messamer, P. (2014). Best practices for incorporating non-aphasia-specific apps into therapy. *Seminars in Speech and Language, 35*, 17–24.

Rochon, E., Laird, L., Bose, A. & Scofield, J. (2005). Mapping therapy for sentence production impairments in nonfluent aphasia. *Neuropsychological Rehabilitation, 15*, 1–36.

Ross, K. B. & Wertz, R. T. R. (1999). Comparison of impairment and disability measures for assessing severity of, and improvement in, aphasia. *Aphasiology, 13*, 113–124.

Saffran, E. M. & Martin, N. (1990). Effects of syntactic priming on sentence production in an agrammatic aphasic. Paper presented at the 28th Annual Meeting of the Academy of Aphasia, Baltimore, MD.

Saffran, E. M., Berndt, R. S. & Schwartz, M. F. (1989). The quantitative analysis of agrammatic production: Procedure and data. *Brain and Language, 37*, 440–479.

Schwartz, M., Linebarger, M. & Saffran, E. M. (1985). The status of the syntactic theory of agrammatism. In M.-L. Kean (Ed.), *Agrammatism*. New York: Academic Press.

Schwartz, M. F., Linebarger, M., Brooks, R. & Bartlett, M. R. (2007). Combining assistive technology with conversation groups in long-term rehabilitation for aphasia. Moss Rehabilitation Research Institute. Retrieved from http://www.researchgate.net/publication/228999447_Combining_assistive_technology_with_conversation_groups_in_long-term_rehabilitation_for_aphasia

Schwartz, M. F., Saffran, E. M., Fink, R. B., Myers, J. L. & Martin, N. (1994). Mapping therapy: A treatment programme for agrammatism. *Aphasiology, 8*, 19–54.

SentenceShaper®. (2015). http://www.sentenceshaper.com

Shankweiler, D., Crain, S., Gorrell, P. & Tuller, B. (1988). Reception of language in Broca's aphasia. *Language and Cognitive Processes, 4*, 1–33.

Sights 'n Sounds 2. (2015). Retrieved from http://www.bungalowsoftware com/sights2. htm

Siri: Your personal assistant. (2009). http://www.siri.com

Slobin, D. I. (1996). From "thought and language" to "thinking for speaking". In J. Gumperz & S. Levinson (Eds.), *Rethinking linguistic relativity*. Cambridge: Cambridge University Press.

The EVA Project. (2015). Retrieved from http://smcse.city.ac.uk/eva/

Thompson, C. K., Choy, J. J., Holland, A. & Cole, R. (2010). Sentactics®: Computer-automated treatment of underlying forms. *Aphasiology, 24*, 1242–1266.

TouchSpeak. (2015). Retrieved from http://www.touchspeak.co.uk/.

True, G., Bartlett, M. R., Fink, R. B., Linebarger, M. C. & Schwartz, M. (2010). Perspectives of persons with aphasia towards SentenceShaper To Go: A qualitative study. *Aphasiology, 24*, 1032–1050.

Video Assisted Speech Technology. (2015). Retrieved from http://www.speakinmotion.com

Weinrich, M., Shelton, J. R., McCall, D. & Cox, D. M. (1997). Generalization from single sentence to multisentence production in severely aphasic patients. *Brain and Language, 58*, 327–352.

Wilson, S., Roper, A., Marshall, J., Galliers, J., Devane, N., Booth, T. & Woolf, C. (2015). Codesign for people with aphasia through tangible design languages. *CoDesign, International Journal of CoCreation in Design and the Arts.*

wordQ+speakQ. (2015). Retrieved from http://www.goqsoftware.com/wordQspeakQ. php

Write:OutLoud®. (2015). Retrieved from http://donjohnston.com/writeoutloud/

Wulfeck, B. B., Bates, E. & Capasso, R. (1991). A cross-linguistic study of grammaticality judgments in aphasia. *Brain and Language, 41*, 311–336.

Deborah Dahl

10 Evaluating speech and language applications for language disorders

Abstract: Chapter 10 discusses evaluation criteria for selecting software that addresses speech and language disorders. It discusses criteria from the point of view of the user as well as from the point of view of someone assisting the user. From the user's perspective, the major considerations are efficacy, time to results, ease of learning, user engagement, quality of feedback, accuracy of speech and language technologies, and usability. From the perspective of someone who is helping the user (such as a parent or clinician) important criteria include cost, support for multiple users, customization, availability of technical support, language support, extensibility, record keeping, assessment tools, ease of administration, and platform support. The chapter concludes by presenting a strategy for selecting and evaluating the software under consideration.

10.1 Use of the software

10.1.1 Some general considerations

Clinicians, end users, and family members will be faced with the problem of choosing software for a particular speech or language disorder. This can be a difficult problem. Family members in particular may have difficulty finding the time to explore all the different software options. No one wants to waste time and money on products that will frustrate users and not produce results, so it is well worth taking the time to carefully evaluate software to make sure that it meets the user's needs.

Since the number of applications that address speech and language disorders is large and continually expanding, it is not possible to provide a definitive list of high-quality applications here. However, we can discuss some criteria to keep in mind while looking at options. We will classify the criteria into those pertaining to direct use of the software and those pertaining to contextual and support features. Some features are essential and others are either simply nice to have or are useful when comparing two otherwise more or less equivalent products. Obviously, the final selection is very likely to involve tradeoffs because no one system is likely to completely satisfy all the user's needs. The person who is selecting products will have to take all of these tradeoffs into account and decide what the best choice is for their situation.

10.1.2 Efficacy

Certainly efficacy is a high priority for any evaluation. Whether it is an assistive product or a remediation product, it has to work. Evaluating efficacy can be difficult, especially for remediation products that work over the long term. Positive outcomes of well-designed, unbiased, peer-reviewed experiments testing efficacy are ideal evidence for efficacy, but these are not always available. Fully documented case studies in peer-reviewed journals are also useful in evaluating efficacy, although not as convincing as experimental studies. This area is unfortunately not very well funded, and it is difficult to get support for efficacy studies, so the lack of efficacy studies for a particular piece of software does not necessarily mean that it does not work. In addition, efficacy studies take a long time to do and to get published, so results from research that is still ongoing may not be available. Finally, end users and family members may not have the background to evaluate technical research literature. Thus, often, it will be necessary to get more indirect evidence for effectiveness.

It is also important to keep in mind that effectiveness is not an all-or-none characteristic. Some products might be less effective than others but may still be effective enough, taking into account other considerations such as cost and user engagement. Here are some questions to ask:

1. Has the software been adopted by well-respected clinicians and/or research centers? If it has been widely used for a long time, that in itself provides good evidence for efficacy. Of course, it is possible that very innovative and effective software is not widely used simply because it is so new, so the lack of widespread use is not necessarily a negative.
2. Evidence for efficacy can also be found, in many cases, by looking at theories underlying a product. Even if a product has not itself been tested in formal experiments, it may be based on a theory that has been tested. White papers summarizing the relevant research literature are often available on product websites, which is useful for people who do not have the time or background to deal with the primary literature.
3. Are positive testimonials and product reviews from clinicians, family members, or end users available? These are especially useful if they are found on the web and not just on the software's website. Are there negative product reviews, and if so, do the negative comments affect critical features of the software or are they more incidental or cosmetic? Videos of the product in use can be useful, but care should be taken in evaluating videos, since the product's vendors will of course not publish a video that would give a negative impression of the product.
4. What are the credentials of the product's designers? Do they have a solid academic background in the relevant field(s)? Certainly, it is possible for effective

software for speech and language disorders to be developed by non-experts, but it is much more likely that credentialed developers with deep expertise in the field will develop an effective product. Since applying speech and language technology to language disorders is interdisciplinary by nature, ideally, the developers should have a background in both the disorders themselves and the speech and language technologies they are using.

10.1.3 Time to results (for remediation software)

Even if the software works, if it takes a long time to see results or improvement is very slow, this may be discouraging for users. Some disorders, by their nature, are likely to show very slow improvement, even with support from the best possible software, so there may be no alternative to slow progress, but in general, faster results are to be preferred. Product reviews and testimonials are useful in comparing how long it takes different products to get results.

10.1.4 Learning to use the software

How long does it take to learn to use the software? Is the user interface easy to understand? This is probably best determined by working with an evaluation copy of the software because it is very difficult to evaluate a user interface without hands-on experience. A software product that is difficult to learn will discourage end users and make them less likely to use the software, no matter how effective it is. Difficulty for the end user, of course, is important. But it is also important to take into account the learnability for the clinician, technical support person, or family member who is also working with the software. If the end user has other disabilities in addition to their speech or language disorder, such as cognitive impairments (for example, dementia or Down syndrome) or impairments in sustaining attention (ADHD), then the user interface may need to take those disabilities into account. Similarly, software designed for children may need a simpler user interface than software designed for adults.

10.1.5 User engagement

Is the product engaging? Do users enjoy using it? Are the exercises interesting and attractive for the end user? (It is important to consider these criteria from the point of view of the end user, who is actually going to be using the product, not from the point of view of the purchaser of the product.) If users do not like to use the software, they will use it less and be less likely to develop fluency with the user interface. They may even stop using it altogether. Different people are engaged by different software, so, like learning curve, engagement is best assessed by hands-on experience with a trial version. Product reviews and testimonials can also be helpful here.

10.1.6 Responsiveness/robustness/implementation quality

The product has to meet basic standards of stability and software quality. This is not normally a significant problem with standard products, but may be an issue with cutting-edge software developed by a research institution. Does the system respond quickly enough to keep the user engaged? Does it crash or hang during use? Do any screens fail to lead anywhere? These issues are especially important for software designed for people with disabilities, who may find it difficult to get past software problems that other people might be able to ignore.

Many products for speech and language disorders contain significant multimedia content. If the system includes audio, is it clear and free of noise? Similarly, are any displayed images or graphics crisp and meaningful? Do video and animations play fluently? Is any displayed text clear, with an easy-to-read font size?

10.1.7 Feedback

For remediation software, what kind of feedback does the system provide on the user's inputs? Is the feedback accurate, comprehensible, and helpful? Does the feedback distract the user or interfere with their use of the software? Can the type and frequency of feedback be customized?

10.1.8 Accuracy of speech and language technologies

Speech recognition and natural language understanding are not perfect technologies and may sometimes do the wrong thing. For example, a word may be misrecognized as a different word. Are recognition failures so frequent that they become a distraction or confuse the end user?

10.1.9 Usability in light of other issues

Can the software be used by a user who has physical issues accompanying their speech and language disorders? For example, many people with aphasia have right-side hemiplegia, which makes it difficult to use a mouse or to hold a mobile device in two hands. This consideration is especially important to take into account for assistive technologies, which, in many cases, need to be portable.

10.2 Contextual and support features

The criteria discussed above all had to do with the user's actual use of the software. Now we turn to criteria that will also be important for people who are helping the end user.

10.2.1 Cost, including initial cost and updates/new materials

Cost has to be taken into account. If the software is at all expensive, then it is very important to consider whether the vendor offers a trial or evaluation version. Not only the initial cost should be taken into account, but also the cost of updates for new versions and any new modules with supplementary material. A monthly or yearly subscription model is becoming more common with all kinds of software. If the software is offered as a subscription, then the total cost over the time in which the software will be used has to be considered. In addition, subscription for a month or two can be an alternative to an evaluation version. Note whether the vendor will offer a refund if the software does not meet the user's needs.

10.2.2 Multiple users

If the software will be used by several different users, for example, in a clinic, or in a clinician's office, it should be able to accommodate multiple users, each with their own exercises, treatment goals, and records.

10.2.3 Personalization and customization

How easy is it to personalize the application? In many applications, it is useful for users to be able to personalize the application and the user interface.

Users may want to include personal vocabulary such as their name, the names of family members, or they might wish to include their own pictures, in applications where customized pictures can be used. It is also very useful if exercises can be customized for the user's specific needs.

10.2.4 Support/user community/documentation

What kinds of support options are available? The two most common options are vendor-supplied support and community support, which is becoming much more common for all software. By their nature, user communities for this kind of software may be small, so community support may be limited, simply because there are relatively few users. Vendor-supplied support may also be limited if the vendor is a small organization. If bugs are reported publicly on a message board forum, does the vendor respond to the messages, and are bugs quickly addressed?

For more complex remediation software, is there a community of clinicians who are familiar with the software and who can guide users in at least the initial phases of using it and who can interpret and make use of any record-keeping features?

10.2.5 Languages

It goes without saying that the software needs to support the language(s) of the intended users. Speech and language technologies have been most thoroughly developed for English. If the software is multilingual but it is being purchased for speakers of languages other than English, it is very important to evaluate the quality of the speech and language technologies for the specific language that the users will be speaking. Even if the system works well for English speakers, it may not work well for speakers of other languages.

10.2.6 Extensibility and growth

Especially in the case of remediation software, does the software cover a breadth of issues related to the disorder or does it just focus on one aspect? Is there a range of levels of difficulty, or will the user quickly get to a point where the software is too easy?

10.2.7 Record keeping

Internal tools to keep track of use of the software in terms of overall time spent as well as time spent on specific activities can be helpful, especially for remediation software used in a clinical setting. Software-based record-keeping tools have significant advantages over manual record-keeping in terms of consistency and completeness. Software tools can also do things that would be very difficult to do manually, such as maintaining precise time-stamps of the user's activities. If record-keeping tools are available, do they keep track of enough information?

10.2.8 Assessment

For remediation software, assessment tools to keep track of progress can be useful for the clinician and motivating for the user. If there are assessment tools, how easy are they to use? What kinds of reports do they produce, both for individual sessions as well as for multiple sessions covering different periods?

10.2.9 Administration

If the software can be used by more than one person, for example, in a clinic, how easy is it to add, delete, and modify users? Will the software be used in a context where passwords are appropriate, and if so, is it easy to administer passwords?

10.2.10 Platform – is the product available on convenient, widely available platforms?

The product should be available on at least one widely available platform. Currently, these include Windows or Apple desktop computers, Apple or Android tablets, and Apple or Android phones, running the current versions of their operating systems. In the case of assistive software in particular, it may be important for the software to be portable. If the platform is a tablet or other portable device, is the battery life reasonable so that the user does not have to keep charging the device's batteries?

10.2.11 Evaluation strategy

Overall, the strategy for finding and evaluating software for language disorders should involve the following steps.

1. Understand the user's needs. Do they need assistive technology, remediation technology, or both? Does the software that they will be using need to be very simple to use or can they use a more complex user interface (or will someone be helping them with the user interface)? How important is mobility? How important is record keeping?

2. Take your time and try to review several options if possible. Take advantage of free trial offers. Talk to other people who are addressing the same disorder. Do not forget to look at research software.

3. In evaluating the software, be sure that an actual end user tries it and be sure to test it in the actual environments where it will be used. No one can decide if the software is usable other than the actual end user. Be sure that they spend a reasonable amount of time trying it out before deciding whether or not to get it. If the end user does not like the software or does not seem to want to use it, they can be encouraged to use it, but ultimately, they are not likely to get much benefit from software that they do not want to use or that they avoid using.

11 Conclusions

As the previous chapters have shown, emerging speech and language technologies have great and growing potential for remediating, assessing, and providing assistive technology for people with language disorders. We have explored in detail four specific programs – GrammarTrainer, MossTalk Words, Aphasia Therapy System, and SentenceShaper – and have reviewed many other programs in less detail. At this point, it is worthwhile to step back and discuss several themes.

11.1 Feedback

We return multiple times to the role of feedback. To what extent should software identify, point out, and correct user's errors as opposed to simply trying to grasp the user's intention? In addition, should this be a variable parameter set by a clinician or user, depending on the user's goals in interacting with the software? Our detailed examples take several perspectives on this question. GrammarTrainer and the Aphasia Therapy system provide extensive feedback, MossTalk Words can be set to be more or less strict about the user's productions, and SentenceShaper – which is designed to support and strengthen self-monitoring – will accept anything that users say, assigning them the task of evaluating and modifying their own productions.

11.2 Assistive and remediative goals

We also recognize a tension between assistive and remediative goals. Assistive technology will support the user's overall goal of communicating with others, but many users will also benefit from remediation technologies. Remediation technologies reduce the user's need for assistive technologies by strengthening their own abilities. In some cases, these goals can be addressed by the same software, for example, both SentenceShaper and Lingraphica, discussed in earlier chapters, though originally designed as assistive technologies, have been shown to improve communication after a period of use. Clinicians, family members, and users will have to decide how to balance the relative emphasis on assistive technology and remediation for each user.

11.3 Acquisition and repair

An important difference among the disorders we discuss is between disorders like aphasia, which affect adults with established language ability, and disorders like Specific Language Impairment in children, where language has not yet been fully acquired. Techniques like those used in SentenceShaper, Aphasia Therapy System, and MossTalk help users to access their underlying language ability, while Grammar Trainer focuses on helping its users learn language in the first place.

11.4 Reinforcements/rewards

Another consideration, particularly where remediation software is concerned, is what sorts of reinforcements to offer for correct answers or task completion. Many of the programs for children with language impairments offer short animation sequences of the sort that younger children find rewarding, but which might not be appropriate for older kids or adults. GrammarTrainer is more customizable: upon logging in, the user or supervisor types in the name of an appropriate external reward and the number of points the user needs to accumulate before obtaining it. Rewards, whether built in (as in the case of animations) or external (as with GrammarTrainer), are an essential part of successful training, motivating users to expend the time and energy necessary for progress. Adults with acquired aphasia may need less explicit motivation because they are to some degree already motivated by their interest in improving their language skills.

11.5 Next steps

Improvements in the basic technologies are key. Speech recognition for people with speech and language disorders is still not as accurate as speech recognition for the general population. Although it is sufficiently accurate for many applications, more accurate recognition would reduce the need for speaker-dependent training and reduce frustration for users. More accurate recognition would also make it possible to add productive speech training to the various programs that teach productive language to language-impaired children. These programs currently only accept text-based input from users; allowing speech input not only provides more robust training in productive language, but also expands access to users who struggle with printed word recognition. And, since most people can speak faster than they can create text, speech input options would also speed up training and reduce some of its more tedious and potentially distracting aspects.

Although speech recognition of words is relatively well advanced, processing intonation (prosody) is still a research topic. Easy-to-use software for prosodic analysis would be very helpful in building applications for users with abnormal prosody. It might also enable text-to-speech devices to add such punctuation marks as periods and commas, which are often associated with particular intonation patterns.

Related to the general theme of balancing remediation goals and assistive goals, speech recognizer parameters such as confidence should be easy to control, allowing systems to be more or less strict about the inputs they will accept, depending on particular users and goals.

Although software tools for incorporating existing speech and language technologies into other systems' Application Programming Interfaces, or APIs, are becoming easier to use, using these tools, and creating good user interfaces for these applications, still requires significant expertise and is often difficult for average developers to master. These tools need to be easier to use.

Research on efficacy and usability of software for language disorders needs greater support. The perceived small market size for applications for people with speech and language disorders makes it unlikely that large companies will invest in these types of applications. This small market also makes it difficult for startups to convince investors that a product is worth investing in. On the other hand, funding agencies often perceive software development and efficacy testing as a commercial activity, which again, leads to a lack of funding in these areas. Consequently, it is very easy for software to be developed and marketed with no more than, at best, anecdotal evidence that it is effective. Ineffective software is not only a waste of money, but more importantly, it wastes both the user's time and the time of family members who may be helping the user.

We hope that this book has proven to be valuable to all our audiences: developers who are interested in creating applications that use speech and language technologies to address language disorders; clinicians who would like to use these technologies with their clients; students of speech and language therapy; and finally, the end users and their family members, who are looking for ways to reduce the often devastating impact that language disorders can have on their lives.

Authors' biographies

Katharine Beals specializes in the educational and linguistic needs of children with autism and other language delays. She is an adjunct professor at the Drexel University School of Education, having designed two of the five classes for Drexel's Graduate Certificate in Autism Spectrum Disorders. She is also a lecturer at the University of Pennsylvania Graduate School of Education, teaching courses on autism and language delays. And she is the designer of the GrammarTrainer software program, discussed in Chapter 4. She received a PhD in linguistics from the University of Chicago in 1995 and worked for 5 years in the Natural Language Group at Unisys Corporation. Her articles on the educational needs of children with autism and language delays have appeared on *TheAtlantic.com*, *Education Next*, and *Education News*. She has also written on technology for autism, most recently contributing a chapter to *Technology Tools for Children with Autism*. She is the author of *Raising a Left-Brain Child in a Right-Brain World: Strategies for Helping Bright, Quirky, Socially Awkward Children to Thrive at Home and at School*.

Deborah Dahl is a consultant in speech and natural language technologies. She received a PhD in linguistics from the University of Minnesota in 1984 and was a post-doctoral fellow in Cognitive Science at the University of Pennsylvania from 1983 to 1984. Following her post-doctoral work, Dr. Dahl developed natural language understanding technology at Unisys Corporation and integrated natural language systems with speech recognition for both government and commercial applications. She has been an independent consultant since 2002 and has specialized in applications of speech and natural language technology for both the general population and for users with disabilities. Dr. Dahl implemented the speech recognition feature of MossTalk Words described in Chapter 8 and participated in the development of the natural language understanding technology used in the Aphasia Therapy System described in Chapter 9. She is an active participant in international standards for multimodal interaction and for web accessibility for people with cognitive disabilities at the World Wide Web Consortium. She is the editor of the book *Practical Spoken Dialog Systems*. Dr. Dahl is a regular columnist in *Speech Technology Magazine* and has twice received the Speech Luminary award from *Speech Technology Magazine* for contributions to the speech industry.

Ruth Fink, MA, CCC-SLP, is the clinical director of MossRehab Aphasia Center and a senior staff research associate of Moss Rehabilitation Research Institute. She has been treating adults with aphasia in various settings since 1969. In 1989, she joined the staff of Moss Rehabilitation Research Institute and began to conduct aphasia research under the mentorship of Dr. Myrna Schwartz. As a research speech-language pathologist she has extensive experience in the design and implementation of single subject and small group treatment experiments with aphasic adults. She has served as co-Principal Investigator and project director on both single-site and multisite treatment studies, including federally funded treatment grants in the areas of sentence processing disorders, word retrieval disorders, and computer-assisted applications. Her work has appeared in such publications as *Aphasiology, Clinical Aphasiology, Brain and Language, American Journal of Speech-Language Pathology, Neuropsychological Rehabilitation, Topics in Stroke Rehabilitation, American Speech-Language Hearing Association Newsletter, Journal of International Neuropsychological Society,* and *Behavioral Neurology and Neuropsychology.* She has also presented her work at the American Speech-Language Hearing Association Convention, the Academy of Aphasia, and Clinical Aphasiology Conference. In addition to her work in MRRI, Ms. Fink is a member of the American Speech Language Hearing Association, a Special Interest Division 2 (SID 2) affiliate of Neurophysiology and Neurogenic Speech and Language Disorders, and a member of the Academy of Aphasia. She earned an MA at Temple University and a BA at Montclair State College, both in speech-language pathology.

Among her proudest achievements are her contribution to the development and dissemination of MossTalk Words software and her role in co-founding and growing the MossRehab Aphasia Center, a warm and supportive environment that offers opportunities for individuals with aphasia to participate in research, cutting-edge treatments, and supportive activities to enhance their quality of life, including book clubs, conversation groups, and computer laboratories.

Marcia Linebarger's professional life has revolved around three disciplines: formal linguistics, the study of acquired language disorders, and the development of computer software. She received a PhD in linguistics from Massachusetts Institute of Technology in 1980, writing her dissertation on the syntax and semantics of negative polarity. She completed postdoctoral training in aphasiology at the University of Pennsylvania, exploring language processing in aphasia with Myrna Schwartz (Moss Rehabilitation Research Institute) and Eleanor Saffran (Temple University). In 1985, she entered the field of computational linguistics, developing natural language understanding technology at Unisys Corporation. Ten years into this position, she was able to join these varied professional threads when she received a grant from NIDCD to develop aphasia treatment software at Unisys and investigate its effects at MossRehab with her former colleagues. During this grant, Dr. Linebarger invented SentenceShaper®, a communication aid for aphasia. Research studies with the program were quite promising, and in 2001, she left Unisys and started her own small business, Psycholinguistic

Technologies, Inc., which has released SentenceShaper as a commercial product. In subsequent NIH-funded collaborations between Psycholinguistic Technologies and MossRehab (Myrna Schwartz) and the University of Maryland (Rita Berndt, Denise McCall), she examined the impact of SentenceShaper as a communication aid and as a therapy tool. In recent years, Dr. Linebarger has focused upon further developing the software and provides computer coaching for people with aphasia to help them make use of SentenceShaper and other appropriate technology.

Index

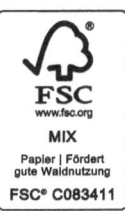

MIX

Papier | Fördert
gute Waldnutzung

FSC® C083411

Zeitfracht Medien GmbH
Ferdinand-Jühlke-Straße 7
99095 Erfurt, Deutschland
produktsicherheit@kolibri360.de